Girl on the Net

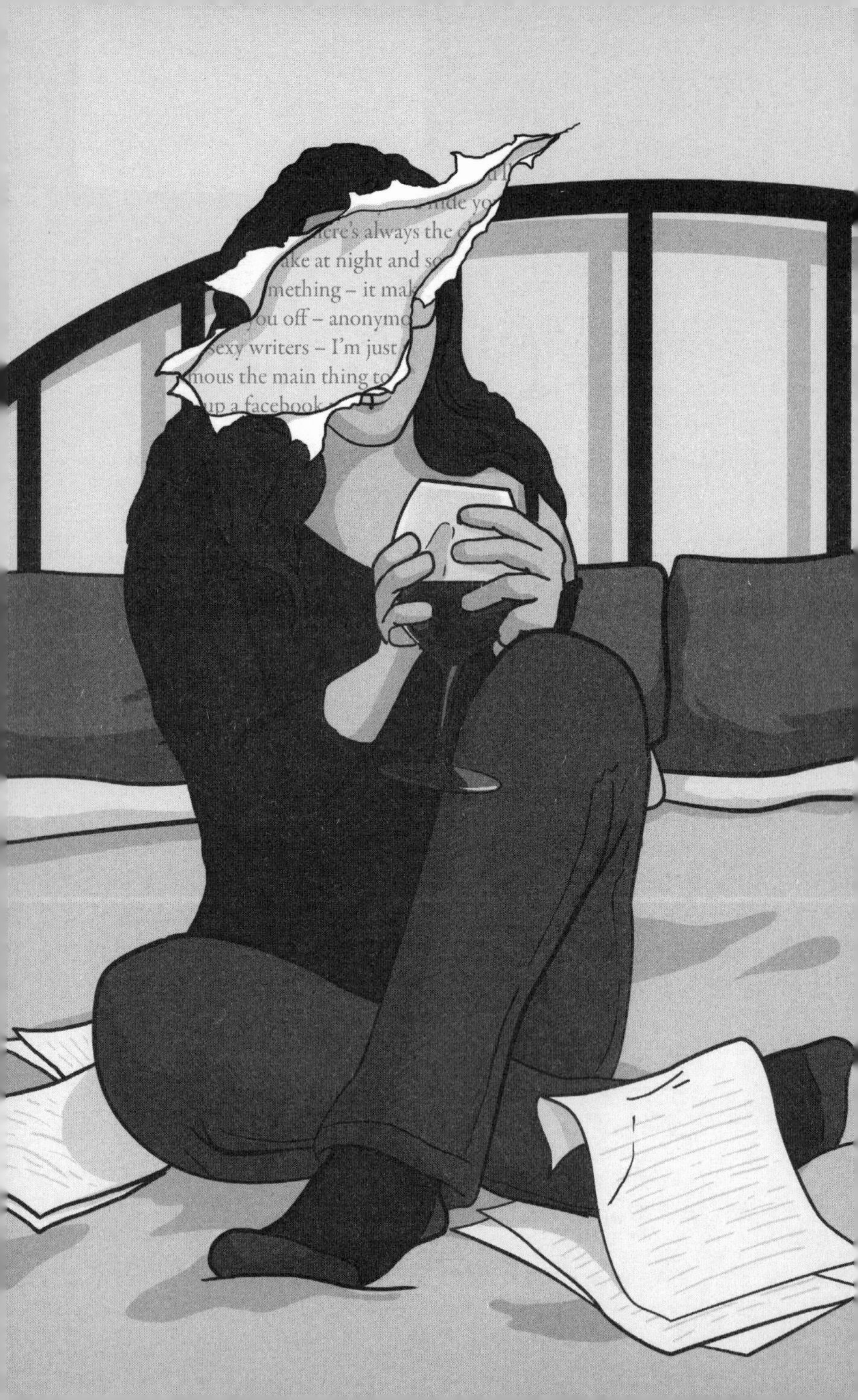
here's always the
ake at night and so
mething – it mak
you off – anonymo
sexy writers – I'm just
mous the main thing to
up a facebook

Girl on the Net

how a bad girl fell in love

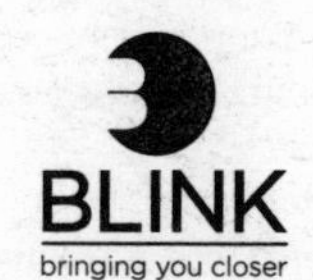

Published by Blink Publishing
3.25, The Plaza,
535 Kings Road,
Chelsea Harbour,
London, SW10 0SZ

www.blinkpublishing.co.uk

facebook.com/blinkpublishing
twitter.com/blinkpublishing

PB – 978-1-910536-57-5

A CIP catalogue of this book is available from the British Library.

Cover design by Emily Rough, Blink Publishing
Typeset by www.envydesign.co.uk

Printed and bound by Clays Ltd, St Ives Plc

1 3 5 7 9 10 8 6 4 2

Papers used by Blink Publishing are natural, recyclable products made from wood grown in sustainable forests. The manufacturing processes conform to the environmental regulations of the country of origin.

Blink Publishing is an imprint of the Bonnier Publishing Group
www.bonnierpublishing.co.uk

Contents

For content notes visit http://www.girlonthenet.com/content.

Introduction

The chapter titles in this book come from genuine advice articles online. When we head to Google to ask those nagging questions (*What is love? How do I know when someone loves me? How do I spice up my sex life? What counts as cheating?*) these articles are all trying to give us an answer. Some give great answers, some give bad. Most fall somewhere in between.

This book is about love, but it's not a love story. It's full of dirty bits, but it's not really porn. It includes some advice, but it's not a self-help book: I'm no more qualified to help you than I'm qualified to fly a plane. It won't give you the answers people hit 'Search' for, but it'll give you some of *my* answers and I'll leave you to work out where I'm wrong.

What is Love? Five Theories On The Greatest Emotion Of All

(*Guardian.com*)

Me (sexy voice): Got a hot surprise for you when you get home.
Him: Is it macaroni cheese?

On a typical morning, I wake up to Radio 4 and the casual prodding of a 7am erection – which as we all know is the hardest kind. Mark – placid nerd and owner of the aforementioned erection – whistles a half-adorable, half-annoying snore as he wraps me in a big, warm, hug. He smells promisingly like the lazy sex we had the night before, which gives me a brief kick of arousal. There's no time to explore that though, because it's Wednesday – a work day – and we have to get up. I wander into the kitchen and pour coffee beans into a brushed aluminium coffee grinder. Birds sing, neighbours clatter through the flat upstairs getting ready for work and just as the kettle starts to boil I hear the comforting pad of Mark's feet as he lumbers along the hallway. Looking sleepily wrinkled from the pillow, he murmurs: 'Coffee? I love you so much.'

It's at this point that I wonder – what the tedious suburban *fuck* has happened to my life?

A few years ago my typical Wednesday would start with a weird taste in my mouth and the awkward moment where I would try and remember if I'd developed a skin condition or if that really *is* dried spunk on my forearm. The kind of day that begins with a sniff of promise – like the guy next to me in bed might turn out to have a fascinating fetish and a flat with its own dungeon, or he could be the kind of fuckbuddy who'll send a text at lunchtime promising post-work beers and a hand job. Five years ago there was no such thing as a typical Wednesday for me. It could have been spent with a guy I was casually shagging, bitching about work until the end of exactly two pints, before tripping off to his flat to have messy, easy sex on his perfectly made bed. It could have been a date with a stranger, revelling in that flutter of horny excitement when you realise that this one lives up to the grand promises he made on *PlentyOfFucks.com*, or wherever he hailed from. Maybe something less sex-oriented: dinner, karaoke, comedy, cocktails. Perhaps the odd night in to recharge and swap diary dates with a guy dropping in from out of town.

But these days, Wednesdays are all 'Did you fill out the mortgage paperwork?' and 'Is your mum coming to visit this weekend?' and maybe 'As a special treat let's get a takeaway this evening while we watch *Game of Thrones*'.

What happened to me? Where did my adventure go? Why am I *hand-grinding* coffee, for Christ's sake?

You might be thinking right now that this kind of tranquil loved-up morning seems right up your alley – comfort, security and no need to go through the terrifying rigmarole of chatting people up before you get to rummage in their trousers. But if, on the other hand, you've spent most of your life chasing that stomach-tingling kick of lust when a new person puts their hand up your shirt, you may well wonder why anyone would choose to swap that for a sexless morning hug and a TV box set or two.

I'm a sex blogger. While most people who hear that go 'Oh, like *Belle de Jour*?' sadly I'm not even half as cool as she is and nor do I make money from shagging. I doubt I'd make much with my incompetent seduction anyway, even if I threw in Tesco Clubcard points. I'm more like a sex trainspotter: chasing a whole bunch of hot experiences then documenting them in drooling, excitable detail for the titillation of people on the Internet. The blog started as a nifty way to tell filthy stories about the guys and girls I'd shagged, without boring my friends in the pub about all the different ways you can milk a prostate. If I'm honest, I also wanted to rage against the idea that women don't really want sex: that only men or dogs feel genuine, aching lust. While I was keen to be able to boast about the time I got to have a threesome with two guys, I was even keener to confront the weird notion that women who enjoy sex are like unicorns – only rarer and with fewer legs.

So far, so totally average: girl has a lot of sex with a bunch of different people, writes about it on the Internet, drinks gin, has a wank, finds more sex partners. The cycle continues until either she dies, or something equally calamitous happens.

My calamity is called Mark: the guy with the excessive coffee enthusiasm and rock-hard morning boner. Mark is the 26th guy I ever fucked, and if it sounds creepy that I know the exact number, I refer you to the point above about sex blogging. When I started writing stories about the people I'd been with, it felt important to maintain a degree of consistency. At the very least, I wanted to get everything in the right order. So: Mark. Number 26. Nerdy, hot, tall, broad and pretty keen on the rituals involved in making a truly wank-worthy cup of coffee. Those aren't his best features, by the way, but it's hard to identify what his best features are because he just seems to draw love out of me via a baffling romantic osmosis.

Mark reminds me of a character from *Dr Who*: Rory, the boyfriend of one of the Doctor's assistants. Rory is a clumsy boy-next-door, and is initially written off by most other characters as someone who sits in the background. He's not a smouldering, distant lover or a knight in shining armour, and if he had a superpower it would be patience. In the show, Rory's girlfriend, Amy, gets to go on the adventures, have all the lines and occasionally kick ass. The magic of Rory is in the fact that no matter what Amy does, or who she meets, she cannot help but love him. Likewise with Mark: he isn't a secret billionaire or a tortured artist or a guy with a dark secret that only love can help unravel; he is just there – doing small, everyday, amazingly sexy things. Sometimes it's the gentle way he tucks me into bed when I'm shattered and on the verge of crying. Other times it's the sight of him frowning in concentration at a computer screen, idly eating buttered crumpets, or the way he – in a softly Mancunian accent – pronounces 'buttered crumpets'. There are his big arms and his creative swearing. And, let's not forget – because I haven't become a *completely* saccharine arsehole – occasionally his best feature is his cock.

So we've established that I love Mark. But, if you're currently single and wanting to push my smug arse off the nearest bridge, please don't panic. There's a reason I'm starting the story here.

Most romances seem to end in a dreamlike 'happy ever after' like this one. Our protagonist has lugged a pile of baggage up the mountain of dating and eventually planted their flag at the summit. They've swapped uncertainty for security, variety for monogamy, and hand jobs for hand-ground coffee. It sounds nice enough, until you realise that a 'happy ever after' is no more real than the unicorn we met a few paragraphs ago. Life is long, and full of complications, which don't just stop when you find someone lovely; so what the hell do we do between 'happy ever after' and 'the end'? Do we all sit in stasis for 50-odd years when we reach peak suburban bliss? Of course not. In the journey of love and life, we've not climbed the final mountain, just one of many hills – there are still hundreds more of the bastards to scale before we get to have a sit down and a pint. In between falling in love and the sweet release of death we've got everything else to play for: we still fuck, we still fight, we still *live*.

Yet for some reason this myth – that life consists of a series of steps towards the lofty summit of happiness, from which other couples look down on us and urge us on to the next checkpoint – persists: 'when are you getting married?' or 'you simply *must* have children, they'll give your life meaning!' Whether it's family gatherings where people nudge you to pop the question, friends who tell you you'll 'change your mind' about kids, or the *Daily Mail* printing a giant picture of an *actual clock* to remind you that your ovaries will turn to sand if you don't start using them.

The fiction that everyone's happiness can be guaranteed by identical things is not nearly as fun as the truth: we're all beautifully different, and the same choices just won't work for everyone. But while it's easy to say 'I'm not the marrying type', it's far harder to work out just what type I actually am. A horny sex blogger, who can't resist chasing the next shag? Mark's loyal, snuggling sofa companion? A bit of both? Neither?

Standing in the kitchen, hand-grinding coffee, it feels like I'm near the summit of the next mountain. But the only way I want to go is down.

When Mark and I have drunk our coffee, showered and dressed, it's time for our most important morning ritual. I begin it with some surreptitious muttering and a few creative swear words. Mark picks up his cue:

'OK, Sarah, I'll give you ten seconds to have a little panic about this, then I'm going to ring your fucking phone and it'll turn out it's in your bag like it *always* bloody is, because you're a bellend.'

Please don't be alarmed by the swearing. It's taken Mark a long time to start declaring his love through swear words and I never ever want him to stop. We swear and curse because, while he's got an idea of romance as defined by Hallmark, I can't deal with the squishy stuff. When we first got together he'd tell me I was 'great' and I'd have a split second in which to decide what to say. Do I reciprocate? God no – then we'd become one of those couples that spends hours whispering sweet nothings and refusing to put the phone down.

'I love you.'

'I love you *more*.'

'No, I love *you* more...'

...Continue until everyone vomits and we have to spend our weekend deep-cleaning the carpets.

Do I just say 'thank you' and accept the compliment? I'd love to be able to do that, but I'm British, so accepting a compliment essentially constitutes boasting. Shudder. I could deal with the 'you're great' conundrum by denying it utterly, as if the very accusation is slanderous, or asking 'why?' like a petulant child who doesn't understand how reciprocal conversation works. Neither of these methods are particularly fun for Mark, especially because when I put him on the spot with 'why' he can't think of anything great except 'umm... tits?'

So I go with the response that comes most naturally to me: I tell him to fuck off.

It sounds harsh, but 'fuck off' conveys a number of different things: from 'I love you' to 'thanks' to 'come here' as well as – yes – plain 'fuck off'. It's the Swiss army knife of loving conversation. In this instance, when Mark's holding his phone and getting ready to dial mine – thumb hovering over the button that'll shortly expose me yet again as a panicking eejit, 'fuck off' means 'I hope you continue to find me adorable even though I irritate the shit out of you'. Problem is, Mark refuses to accept that all the things he mistakenly believes are my flaws are actually just a trick of his mind. No matter how many times I've hunted for my phone and found it somewhere *other* than my bag – the sofa, the bathroom, his jacket pocket – he'll only remember the times when it was *actually* in my bag, and I spent a stressful ten minutes hurling books and clothes around the flat and accusing him of deliberately hiding my stuff. Naturally, this *one isolated time*, it turns out my phone actually is in my bag, so I have to put up with him being smug for the best part of an hour-long commute while I mutter 'dickhead' under my breath.

I grew up in a very sweary family. We were – and still are – more likely to express love via carefully honed insults than cute cards or unnecessary cuddles. Goodbye hugs happen, but while the act means 'I'll miss you', we're more likely to say 'Thank Christ you're leaving, you tedious old git'.

Occasionally alarmed by our casual rudeness, my mum tries valiantly to sprinkle praise into our conversations: 'You're brilliant, my children. All of my children are *fucking* brilliant,' she'll slur after one too many gin and tonics, bopping her head to whatever tuneless crap someone's bashing out on the piano. 'I'm lucky lucky lucky to have such wonderful children.' Her wonderful children usually reply: 'You would say that, you're pissed.' It sounds obnoxious, like those guys who think 'banter' is the height of wit, but there's nothing I can do about it – it's too deeply ingrained.

Given my upbringing, I'm not sure I could spend the rest of my life with someone who didn't know how to express affection through swearing. The constant barrage of loveliness would feel like being trapped in a kids' TV show. And by embracing my squeamishness about conventional romance, Mark's developed an uncanny knack for backhanded compliments. In his skilled hands, 'you look lovely' can be effortlessly twinned with 'given what you've got to work with', and his winning smile says he only means the first part. It feels closer than the nice words and gentle hugs you'd give to a casual acquaintance. You can say 'I love you' to anyone without fear of hurting their feelings, but you know you're truly treasured if someone calls you a cunt while you cuddle.

I learned all of this from my mum, because although I inherited her foul mouth and excessive love of gin, she also happens to be The Best. Like most mums, she's pretty free with strange advice (any emotional turmoil boils down to 'the weather' or 'your hormones') but her own relationships and heartbreaks taught me more about love than anyone else ever could. She ticked off all the 'happy ever after' boxes pretty early in life with my dad – they got together young, married quickly, had three children before she was 25. But in an exciting twist she fell madly in love with someone else, and decided that a divorce would be better than pretending.

The break hit my dad pretty hard. Not only did he adore Mum, he's also a traditional family man. Some people dream of being rich, others want true love: my dad wanted Sunday afternoon walks and children he could read stories to. His dreams were colourful and picture book – camping holidays in Devon, for instance, where we'd sing 'Waltzing Matilda' around the campfire and thank Daddy for making us a rope swing. Unfortunately real life didn't quite work out like that: the children didn't sit around the hearth waiting patiently for Daddy to come home – we screamed and ran and watched TV and scowled at the thought of learning to read maps. We refused to sit still in the back of the car, or participate in a show-off family sing-along around the tree at Christmas. Our beach trips would be fractured and hectic, with Mum sulking because she hated the outdoors, and Dad howling rage at the smallest child because *of course* you can carry a windbreak, you're three-years-old now, just buck your ideas up.

I've never asked my dad if he felt ripped off. After all, if your dream is love, or money, you can always try again when you get dumped or your hedge fund collapses. With family, though, you're kind of stuck with it. Dad relished the obvious chores of dadhood – vomiting five-year-olds smearing gunk on you in the middle of the night, or needing to wee ten minutes into a car journey. But I wonder if the reality of family *fun* disappointed him a bit. One weekend, we, his eager children, all joined the sailing club, making him burst with pride. But the pride lasted all of five minutes when it became clear we were only interested in pushing the boats as far out into the water as possible, before deliberately capsizing them into the muddy creek. Dad's fantasies of our childhood as one long daddy-led nature walk were often crushed by one or other of us whining that it was too far. It wasn't *fun*. Daddy why must you be so bloody *boring*?

But while it was obvious, even to an eight-year-old, that my parents were very different people, it would never have occurred to me to consider whether they were in love. Had you asked, I would have answered that *of course* they are: they're married, aren't they? Mum and Dad did all the things you'd expect: saying 'I love you' and holding hands and swapping jewellery and watches at Christmas. My dad even bought Mum flowers and took her out to special 'dos' at his work – we'd line up next to the babysitter to bid them goodnight and they looked utterly dazzling. He wore shiny uniforms, had neat hair and opened doors for her, and she wore frothy evening gowns and smiled at him and straightened the collar on his neatly pressed dress shirt – *of course* they were in love.

So when they suddenly announced that they *weren't*, it didn't make much sense. They didn't seem to behave that differently: they still talked and fought and smiled like they'd done before. Dad still took us on walks; Mum still took us to Sainsbury's and told us off for fighting over the last slice of Vienetta. They hadn't really changed as far as I knew and besides, they'd already had their 'happy ever after'! They'd got married and walked off into the sunset! What's marriage, after all, but two people getting together and saying 'Hey, this seems OK, let's keep doing it until one of us dies'. Neither of them had died and he still got her flowers, so what exactly was missing?

Ten years later, when I was 18-years-old and my mum was with my stepdad – the guy she'd left my dad for (rather scandalously not married to him, despite having been together for years), I finally worked out what it was.

At about 11:30 on one of countless Friday nights, I rolled in from the pub, half-pissed and ready to stumble up to bed. Before I collapsed, I popped my head round the door of the dining room to say goodnight to my mum and stepdad. There's music blaring from the stereo and the sound of someone hammering away at a piano.

'An aMAYzing, FEEling, COOOOMing THROUUUUGH...' slurs my stepdad.

'I was BORN to LO-OVE you...' adds my mum. They're both rolling – heads lolling merrily on their necks as they bop along to the song, teeth stained black by cheap supermarket

Rioja. The stereo is cranked up just loud enough that their teenaged children will bang on the walls, and the ancient piano adds some off-key accompaniment for good measure.

'With EEEEvery single beat of my heart.'

She leans on his shoulders, standing behind him and squinting at the lyrics on the disintegrating songbook. He leans forward, flicking his eyes from score to hands and back again as he tries to bash out the chords in time to Freddy's version on the stereo. He fails.

'WO-oh-oh-oh I was BORN to TAKE CARE of youuuuu,' she turns the page of the book and they both go back to squinting.

'EEEEEvery single DAY of my...' They're now focusing so hard on staying upright, it takes them a while to realise that...

'You've turned two pages, you wanker.'

They collapse with laughter, and both reach for their wine.

See what I mean about love? That's why it feels much easier for me to call someone a 'dick' than a 'darling' – the earnest, soft focus kind of love feels less real than the kind that jokes around in the pub, flicking ketchup packets at each other. Or, in Mark's case, editing my name in his phone's address book so I'm stored as 'that forgetful nobhead'.

My parents had that traditional love. I don't want to write off what they had – my mum would kill me if I didn't make it clear that when they first got married she *adored* him. Aching, youthful, true-true love of the kind that has you doodling hearts in a notepad and sobbing with the sheer weight of it. But things changed and the love faded. By the time they divorced, their relationship still looked solid from the outside: a 'happy ever after' learnt from books and films and the traditions their parents had told them were important. Marriage. Children. Sunday walks. Anniversary gifts. Flowers. An *electric* coffee grinder. It can work for some people, if the love is still there, but this one ended because there was nothing behind those tokens. No matter how much you try to fit the template, if the love's not there it won't work – just as putting on a uniform doesn't make you a qualified pilot.

13 Scientifically Proven Signs You're In Love

(*livescience.com*)

Him: I like you. With you I can do all the things I used to wank about.

Let's get back to that Wednesday with Mark. After work, we head to a wine bar that serves 20 different kinds of cheese, because now that we're reasonably settled, fondue has replaced adventure as our evening activity of choice. Outside the bar, we smoke and flirt like we're still 16, and he forgets to take his hand off my arse when my friend Claire arrives.

'Sorry I'm late,' she says, and holds out her phone. 'Want to see a Tinder message from a guy who sculpts fruit?'

Mark, with his straightest face, tells her 'It's all I've ever wanted.'

Claire is newly single. She's already done the marriage thing, but it turned out that her 'Mr Right' was actually just

Mr 'Christ He'll Do I'm Pushing 30', and after a crashing disappointment she's separated and back to what she'd consider Square One: dating. Claire's on a variety of dating sites, where consultants, hipsters, accountants and pricks all compete for her time and attention. She juggles cocktails in the city, cock pictures in her inbox, and her laundry three times a week to keep her bedsheets free from jizz. If I'm honest, it makes me nostalgic.

Claire shows us some messages from Fruit Man and I spend 20 minutes trying to persuade her to reply.

'No,' she makes a face. 'Because then I will be the girl who goes out with a fruit sculptor, and I will never hear the end of it.'

'On the other hand, you'd have the *best* buffet at your wedding reception.'

Claire sighs and scrolls away from a surprisingly well-executed melon ball poodle, through to a few more guys on Tinder. She gives us the highlights as she goes: this one's got a lovely cock. This is the one who made proper breakfast the morning after. This one annoyed her flatmate, but in a hilarious way, so maybe she likes him.

'What about this one?'

'Too boring. Doesn't laugh at my jokes.' There's a short pause before Mark offers: 'Maybe your jokes aren't funny?' And she, in time-honoured tradition, calls him a prick. In case it's not obvious, we love Claire. While I drool over her latest suitor, Mark sits peacefully at one end of the table, playing cartoon games on his iPhone. That's his way. Always nervous of conversation, he'll hide in a corner and occasionally chip in to tell us that he's Googled the row we were having ten minutes ago, and he is ready to announce The Winner.

This time, his main contribution to the conversation comes in the form of a snorted 'bollocks' as Claire informs us both that she's gone off men and has decided to be single for a while.

'Why bollocks?'

'You say that every time we hang out. Then an hour later you think you've been single for long enough.'

Claire laughs, calls Mark something awful, then accepts what he rather gracefully offered as a cue. 'I think I *am* ready for a relationship now though...'

We discuss the options and Claire's ideal man: not too boring, not too wild. Not a sculptor of any food products, despite – and I thought this was worth at least *considering* – his potential to hand-carve sex toys from whatever she had in the veg box. Someone who wants the same things she does. Someone who shares at least one of her passions. They don't necessarily need to be excellent at it, but they need to be willing to try.

'Look at our married friends – they all have their shared passions. Lucy, for instance...'

Lucy and her husband fill their time with crafting, DIY and a million other things you'd only catch me doing for a wage: upcycling and painting and making tables out of wooden crates that they've liberated from the dump. Getting out of bed at 8am on Saturdays to visit car boot sales on the outskirts of London, then cycling ten miles with panniers full of rusting, potential-filled crap.

'Nightmare.'

'Obviously,' Claire agrees. 'The only way you'll find me at a morning car boot sale is if you dumped me there, drunk, the night before. But the point is that they *share* something they love.'

'Are you jealous?'

'Yep. You?'

'Yes. But...' Mark waves away the bottle as I try to pour the wine and smirks because he knows the rant I'm about to launch into. 'I'm not jealous that she's married, or "secure", or any of that bollocks. I'm jealous that she gets a free pass on one of those parent questions. No one's going to nag her about when she'll get married, because she's done it already. She's like the girl who did all her homework on Friday night and has the whole weekend left to play.'

'True,' says Claire. 'I'm still waiting for the "when are you getting married?" nagging to start again in light of the separation. I'm like the girl who did her homework on Friday, then the dog *literally* ate it and now I have to start all over. And this time I want a nice guy to help me with the answers. While we hold hands.'

There's our fundamental difference; I think – to Claire, marriage represents something desirable because it's romantic. To me it just feels like a sensible way to shut everyone up.

Mark's been even quieter than usual since the start of the second bottle of wine, but on the train back, he puts his head on my shoulder, stares down my top and asks:

'Do *we* have any shared passions?'

'Sure,' I think for a bit. '*Game of Thrones*.' He pauses briefly before deciding it doesn't count. Outrageously, he declares that *Breaking Bad* doesn't either.

'*Doctor Who*?'

'Nope.'

'*Parks and Rec*?'

'Jesus.'

'*The Walking Dead*.'

'You're a cunt, you know that?'

I know. But it doesn't sound so cutting when he's leaning on me, breathing warmth down my cleavage and firmly gripping the top of my thigh in the way he does when he's casually horny. I list off more TV shows, and he grips harder.

'*Community*?'

'I hate you.'

'*Grand Designs*.'

'Only *you* like that.' He playfully smacks me on the thigh. It stings, deliciously.

'Your taste in telly is shit, so I like to educate you.'

'Name me a shared passion that isn't to do with telly, *then* we'll talk about "education".'

He smacks my arse for good measure as we walk out of the station and in that way informs me that 'smoking' doesn't count as a shared passion either.

When we get home, shivering after the walk, I can still feel the tingle on my butt cheek from his hand. To show that he knows this, Mark smacks me again in the same place and I grin. He lifts my top up and runs freezing cold fingers down my back, sliding his hands neatly into my jeans and down to the crotch of my knickers. As I bury my face in his neck and stick my tongue out to taste him, he whispers filthy demands in my ear: you're going to do this: you'll lie here. You'll take your fucking knickers down and spread your legs for me.

This routine isn't new, it's a finely honed ritual. The first ever time that Mark and I fucked, it was disappointing, despite our mutual eagerness to get naked together. I'd spent the evening admiring his big hands, broad shoulders and the quiet way he'd smile as if to say 'can we?' He was like the sexiest nerd at the school disco, delighted that he'd been invited to dance. I expected him to fuck me with the kind of wild determination that usually follows a long evening's build-up. But instead he was warm, kind, gentle... and slow. 'Lovemaking', like they do in romantic comedies. Sounds lovely, right? Except I don't tend to wank to 'lovely'. That could easily have been our last ever date. Luckily, I wasn't a totally impulsive arsehole and Mark waited patiently for me to ask him for a second go. After a few more dates, a hell of a lot of experimentation, a few conversations about why it's really nice to end a shag with aching muscles and the odd bite mark, we found a much better sexual rhythm: hard, fast, and with occasional damage to the furniture. Mark takes charge and tells me what to do, just as I want him to. He almost always starts by gripping an item of my clothing, tugging on it like it disgusts him, and ordering: 'Off'. While I love the feeling of his hands pawing at me through my top and knickers, Mark prefers the feeling of flesh on flesh. He likes to see me naked and exposed, so he can touch and grab and smack at me, like everything's on offer for him. Tonight he's not in the mood to strip me himself, so he takes a step back and watches me undress, before diving in – all lips and tongue, with a bonus hand roughly cupping my cunt, sliding his fingers inside me while I grind eagerly against him. We're rarely slow – we rush things – like a couple of eager kids grabbing everything in a sweet shop. He was hard within a few seconds of us walking in the door, because we flirted heavily on the journey home and I know his hand stings from the smack on my thigh just as I can still feel the one on my arse. He pushes me down to my knees and tells me to suck him – just enough to make it good and wet. As I spit on his dick, I fold my arms behind my back, willing him to thrust harder – to push it right down to the back of my throat. It's more fun that way: more intense. Like he's so desperate to come he'll fuck my mouth because he can't wait for me to stand and bend over. I'm messy when I do this. All drool and gagging and watery eyes as I look up. His eyes are closed in concentration and his hands are firmly gripping the sides of my head. Not pulling me *onto* him, just holding me as steady as he can. As if my sole purpose is as a warm, wet mouth for him to fuck: exactly how I like it.

In between the hard thrusts, whispered 'good girls' and my own lust for him thudding hard in the pit of my stomach, at that split second before his dick twitches spunk into the back of my throat, I remember that – oh yeah – we *do* have a shared passion after all.

I try to explain it to him as he drifts off to sleep: that love isn't always about getting married and buying flowers, or even doing crafts together. Sometimes love's about fucking like you want to eat each other, or singing Queen songs at a rickety piano.

'Maybe sometimes,' I whisper to Mark, 'being in love could be about sculpting fruit.'

'Mmf? What the fuck are you on about?'

'I'm talking about shared passions, mate. Like, they don't have to just be romantic ones. They can be weird ones or sexy ones.'

'So love can be about fruit sculpture?'

'Yes. Or shagging: maybe that's ours.'

'Our shared passion is... my dick?'

'Maybe.'

And he yawns, rolls over to grab me, and squashes it into the crack of my bottom:

'My dick *is* brilliant.'

I frown, not sure if I'm explaining this right – either that or he's so knackered he's not up for this kind of waffle. We're all taught to aim for the same generic kind of love: stomach butterflies and 'the one'. Settling down, domestic bliss, etc, etc. But that version of romance is a disappointing lie when compared to the far more interesting truth – love can be playful, unique, and sometimes really weird. It's certainly not easily captured in a wedding photo. 'I think, as a general rule,' Mark murmurs, 'taking dick pics at a wedding is frowned upon.'

30 Signs He's In Love With You

(allwomenstalk.com)

Him: I got you some glitter glue.
Me: Why?
Him: They were throwing it away.
Me: But I hate glitter.
Him: Yeah, but you also hate waste!

Like most kids of the 1990s, I wasted more than a few hours of my life ticking boxes on 'Is he really into you?' quizzes that I found in *Just Seventeen* magazine. Apparently option c) 'being willing to paint my toenails' marked a guy out as 'just a good friend', while 'teasing me about my hair' meant he was up for a snog and perhaps a cheeky grope behind the bike sheds. But on the very next page I'd be confronted with a quiz designed for people who already *had* boyfriends and in that one the teasing was a sign of a casual relationship that wouldn't go anywhere special. Being young,

I failed to learn the obvious lesson from this: when it comes to relationship advice, universal answers are usually horseshit. Instead, I took it to mean that if you really wanted true love then somewhere there had to be a sign. Roses, jewellery, an invitation to his nan's 70th birthday: you'll know what I mean because at some point someone will have told you either to comply with it (if you're a man) or (if you're a woman) to plead for it like it's all you've ever wanted.

The first guy I ever went out with (Number One on the 'Spreadsheet Of Guys I Have Sexed') bought me not just one rose but a whole bush. At the time I boasted to all my friends about it, as if the cheesy tokens their own teenage boyfriends had offered paled into insignificance against this spiky potted stick. As it turns out, this lovely gesture was actually a pain in the arse in disguise. Given that I can barely keep a pet rock without losing it down the back of the sofa, getting me a living, photosynthesising plant was probably a bit much. First Boyfriend (FB) was the king of crap presents, though: tasteless porcelain, tacky T-shirts and jewellery that crumbled when you washed your hands. But he was 16, and for a 16-year-old a plant that lasts more than two months is a serious token of commitment. I used to water it proudly each evening after school, then inevitably let my plant-care routine slide in lieu of running to FB's house to get ham-fistedly fingered in his bedroom. As the rose stick shrivelled, I worried that he'd see my plant neglect as a symbol that my love had died too, and panicked that he wouldn't stick his hand down my knickers any more. So I lied.

'How's that rose I bought you?'

'Doing really well! It's so beautiful! Gorgeous flowers!'

'Really? In *December*?'

Still, a rose bush was definitely a step up from other love tokens I'd received. One Valentine's Day, a gawky, 14-year-old version of me was blushingly delighted to find an anonymous card stuffed into my rucksack outside the science labs. I'd never received a genuine Valentine, although naturally I'd swapped jokey ones with girlfriends and pretended I didn't care about boys. As we all gathered around my real card, giggling and whispering, it struck me that this might actually be my worst nightmare. If you ever wore glasses or looked a bit greasy at school then you know the kind: a boy comes up to you and asks you to go out with his mate. You, despite having never met his mate, say 'yeah OK then' and hug yourself in the knowledge that a guy you haven't noticed has nevertheless noticed you. Your happiness lasts for exactly the time it takes the friend to draw breath, before he huffs 'Hahaha, joke!' and runs away.

I was never great with boys. As an adult I've had numerous conversations with men who lament the fact that girls at school had 'the power'. That 'power' being, of course, the illusion of control over any potential sex. The boys would snog us, try to cop a feel of our tits, then go home frustrated that we'd withheld their ultimate prize – a hand job, or a blow job, or sex, depending on your age and how poorly supervised your school discos were. I always find this lament quite odd – straight guys, even with the benefit of hindsight, still seem to genuinely believe that teenage girls wielded power as if we were demi-gods. Like Neo in the *Matrix* realising there is no spoon, they often go a bit pale when they realise that we experienced the same thing: furtive and frustrating fumbles that never ended with what we wanted, because the boys had to run home for tea, or put on a show of not caring in front of their mates. Or because when it came down to it, their public declarations that they'd 'totally finger that slag' were all to nought when they actually got you alone, and they forgot all about the fingering in favour of making you listen to an entire, tedious album by their new favourite band. If you'd told that horny, lonely version of me that I had the power over guys, I'd have pointed you to the aching throb in the pit of my stomach that could only be cured by a boy who was willing to touch me.

The good news is that this time the card was genuine. The bad news: Mr Valentine wasn't a particularly tempting prospect. He was that one guy in the group about whom everyone swapped weird sexual stories. He showed his dick to so-and-so at the bowling alley. He masturbated in the shower after games. He pinged bra straps and grinned to get your attention, and when that didn't work he'd crack out the big guns: kama sutra positions drawn on exercise books with stick men labelled 'me' and 'your mum'. What's more, the card itself wasn't quite what I'd been led to expect on the most romantic day of the year: it contained a poorly written joke about the size of the boy's penis and an invitation to hop aboard. Essentially it was an early prototype of those Tinder messages that contain just a blurry dick pic and a thinly veiled threat. While I'd have leapt at the chance of a snog, a grope, or pretty much anything in between, the idea of having full sex before I'd even had my nipples touched sounded intimidating: like signing up for a paintball fight and being handed an actual gun. Still, popping on my rose-tinted glasses I decided that his directness could be something of a bonus, because we could skip the awkward stages of teenage dating and head straight for the sticky stuff. If his card had asked for a date I'd have run for the hills – what on earth do you say to each other on a *date* at 14? The whole point of being young is that you don't have to make conversation, because you're far too busy getting touched up.

Terrifying though he was it was clear he was the only outlet for my raging teenage lusts. We came up with an excuse to stay behind when our friends went elsewhere and he gave me one of those licking, sucking, desperate snogs that young people are such experts in. I couldn't care less about the lack of emotion, or the card, with its cartoon giant dick drawn on the front. All I cared about in that second was that there was a boy, with his face linked to my face, stealthily running one hand up my jumper to try and get a feel of nipple. When we talk about significant firsts we usually think of the bases: snog (first base), hand job/fingering (second), oral (third), shag (home run). There's apparently some debate about which base is which (I'm a staunch believer that if you upgrade fingering to third then there's nowhere for oral to go). But the details aren't important – for me this moment with Mr Valentine holds more weight than any arbitrary 'base' because it's the first time, outside my own masturbatory exploration, that I felt the gushing lust that comes with a new sexual discovery. Juice soaked through my knickers and, although I feared it'd leave a huge damp circle in the crotch of my jeans, I was damned if I was going to stop before his snaking hand reached my boob. When, after an aching 20 minutes of cunt-throbbing tension, he finally touched nipple (just one, gently – fingers slipped inside my bra and an involuntary high-pitched moan as he felt how taut it was), I nearly screamed with frustration: his success had only made my arousal worse. I'm not sure I expected an orgasm from a grope, but I certainly didn't expect it to just ramp up the horniness further, giving me cramps and almost a limp as I walked home unsated.

As you can see, it's a bit hard to put sex to one side when I'm talking about romance: to me romance has usually been a route to sex, like a Valentine's card with surprise dick joke inside. A love story that doesn't involve the odd knee-trembling grope or sticky-lubed hand job feels as incomplete as breakfast without coffee. Still, while lust can exist outside of other warm emotions (who can honestly say they've never fancied someone they hate?), romantic gestures are designed to signify someone's extra-special importance. You can say 'I love you' with words, but a dirty weekend says 'no, I *really* love you – look how much this cost!' And if you're rose-bush boyfriend, eager to show you're dedicated, then the closest you'll come to that kind of opulence is a romantic night at a Travelodge.

In case you didn't grow up poor and British, a Travelodge is similar to an American motel and they are usually frequented by miserable salesmen and couples having lacklustre affairs. They never have mini bars but occasionally the bored teenager on the reception desk will lend you a corkscrew so you can treat yourself to a cheap bottle of white wine and a very lonely wank. Not the ideal destination for love, but surely you remember being young and having no money? I don't mean desperate poverty, just the low-level inability to buy stuff that we all had before proper jobs were a possibility at the age of 18. Given our small allowances, a night in a Travelodge was pretty damn expensive, even before you factored in the carvery dinner.

We had no money for the bus so First Boyfriend asked his dad to awkwardly chauffeur us to the hotel in his minivan. If I'm honest, I'd have been happier with a tent pitched on some scrubland somewhere for free – we could have had loud, unusual sex without anyone overhearing. But what his idea lacked in thought it made up for in sheer effort: he'd even put rose petals on the bed. Well, not quite rose petals – tiny pink circles made from cardboard and a hole punch.

It was thoughtful, cute and expensive: everything I'd been taught to look out for in a grand romantic gesture. I smiled and nodded and spoke in creepy baby talk about how 'wuvvly' it all was, then later that evening I shut myself in the bathroom and sobbed like a girl who'd been dumped. With my face pressed into a tiny bath towel, I gulped down wails so he wouldn't hear my misery through the door. I wasn't upset because his gesture wasn't good enough: it was everything I'd been told I should want from a guy – effort, preparation, romance. He'd even brought candles, for crying out loud! When I entered the bedroom, my whole body had swelled with pride that somehow, despite my shouty demeanour and greasy hair and awkward geeky glasses, a guy loved me. Yet in the middle of this I was throwing a childish tantrum. Why? Because on the bed of fake petals, he'd only fucked me the once. If this brand of romance is supposed to be what every woman wants, then I'm the most ungrateful girl in the world. It's like a hungry person being presented with a lovely fry-up, then sobbing because they prefer their eggs scrambled.

Most of my romantic stories end like this. Men do lovely things; I spend the evening wondering when the rampant shagging is going to begin; then at some point I cry like a spoiled toddler. A guy I loved at university (number eight if you're still counting) – when I was getting over my shy goth phase and into my 'get drunk then beg guys to fuck me' phase – took me for a Valentine's dinner, complete with cheap Mexican set menu and seemingly endless jugs of margarita. Over our starters we laughed at the other couples in the restaurant, swearing blind we'd never be as boring as they were. During the main course we giggled at how ironic we were having *actual dinner*, when all we wanted to do was fuck. Over dessert we started slurring dirty talk, discussing the sex things we hadn't yet tried and getting odd looks from the nice people on the tables nearby. We licked the plates. We licked each other. We looked like twats. We got the bill. Eventually we staggered home under the weight of burritos and misplaced arrogance, promising fucks that'd make us feel cool again. Then, inevitably, as we lay on the bed he groaned that he was far too full to shag and I pretended to agree. We fell asleep barely touching, and I tried not to cry. When I tell that story today I still make out that the chaste end to the evening was a cute and funny event, that I took in good spirits: 'Hahaha, no of course I didn't mind. I am not *that* pathetic! It definitely didn't break me.' I'm lying, though. In reality I can still feel the waves of hurt sweeping down from my chest, to meet the pulse of arousal coming back up from my crotch. No matter how great any given evening, a voice in my head pokes me with the niggling question: what's the point of romance without sex? What good is Valentine's Day if I end it unfucked?

So go most of my romance stories: candlelit meals and hotel nights either end in a money-shot or a torrent of tears. Gifts are neglected in favour of a shag. I understand the symbolism of a gesture, but I've often struggled with the *point*. I feel like an irritating four-year-old demanding to know why the sky is blue, or why birthdays are nice, or why if you get a Barbie you shouldn't cry and say you'd rather have a truck. Claire would know why, I think: the gestures are good because of what they represent. Flowers mean 'I love you' as sure as '*te amo*' or '*j'adore*' does. And if someone can't tell tedious, argumentative me that they love me with flowers, then what could they possibly do instead?

I'll tell you.

The most romantic thing I ever saw was a kidnap. It wasn't done for me, but god how I wished it was.

Mary loved Simon, and Simon loved Mary – they'd been together nearly two years and he wanted to mark the occasion by doing something special. Mary's idea of special covered a hell of a lot of things I couldn't fathom: silky lingerie, expensive tea sets, cuddly dogs holding hearts that say 'I ruff you!' Despite our differences, Mary and I shared an interest in something far harder to buy in a card shop: spanking. Be it whips, straps, paddles or canes: if you could whack it hard against a naked bottom, chances are we liked it. We'd bonded at a spanking club, lying next to each other with our bums exposed for the headmaster's cane. As I gasped at each harsh crack, itching to reach my hands behind me and massage the pain from my red striped bottom, she put a hand over my mouth, gave me a sparkling smile, and explained 'If you make a fuss, he'll do it harder.' Things like that tend to bind you together, and we'd been good friends ever since.

Her partner, Simon, was my ideal Dom: he combined a certain old-fashioned chivalry with a wicked smile, a generosity of spirit (always the first to get a round in – swoon) and a desire to beat Mary consensually senseless in the bedroom.

For their anniversary, Simon arranged to have Mary kidnapped.

I'm not saying this kidnap was my *ideal* scenario. For a start, the ratios were all wrong. Having more than one kidnap 'victim' was a key part of Mary's fantasy – she and I could act in solidarity, defying the boys and making plans to escape, while secretly enjoying the fact that we couldn't. My role was to initiate these whispers, and create a bit of faux panic, so as three masked men ran into her flat, I could scream like a damsel in distress and help to ramp up the drama. Personally, if a guy I loved was arranging to have hot men throw me in the back of a van, before humping me like I was the last girl on earth, I'd have preferred if he didn't invite my mates. Still, it's what she wanted. Simon ran the plan past me, and I agreed with the kind of enthusiasm you'd usually reserve for free cake.

I did my bit: struggled playfully while they gagged me and threw a black bag over my head. My wrists were cuffed behind my back, and my ankles bound together. The rope was tight enough that I could feel the thud of my pulse against it, but loose enough that I could slip out in an emergency. We – the girls – were dumped in a heap in the back of a dark blue van, and our anonymous captors loomed over us. It's surprising how much you can discern even through a blindfold. One guy was large and stocky, while another had surprisingly delicate fingers. Amidst their muttering, a few echoing footsteps and a whole lot of heavy breathing, I could work out roughly where they were in relation to me, and squirm in just the right way to get a thrill as my bound ankle came into contact with a leather boot.

I knew who the men were, of course, but I tried desperately to forget which was which, so I could fully immerse myself in the fantasy. I focused instead on the physical sensations: hot hands all over me, pinching and smacking: wet lips pressed up against the side of my covered head, my aching need for more slaps and tighter ropes. At one point I recognised a voice, and I thought it may have been Simon, but the accompanying hand yanking up my skirt felt nothing like his. Whoever it was slapped my thigh to make sure he had my attention, and the sting made my stomach throb with a desperate need to be fucked.

'If you want out, drop this,' he commanded, pressing something hard and metallic into my hand. I nodded in frustration, and gripped it so tightly it hurt my wrist. I moaned against the gag, and shifted a bit to try and ruck my skirt up further. If I struggle enough, one of them will fuck me right here in the van, right? Maybe. *Hopefully.*

More struggling.

A different hand pried my thighs apart further, and delivered another stinging slap. A voice – which sounded deep, as if he was deliberately distorting it – told me not to move until we got there. I couldn't ask where, but I pictured woodland. Dark, quiet and dirty. I pictured rope burns from where they'd tie me to a tree. From the smacks on my thigh, I imagined more whacks, this time done with whippy, whittled twigs and branches as they beat me into a sobbing mess. I imagined the sounds I'd choke against the gag as they fucked me in all the ways I wanted them to. I'd go limp like a rag doll, keeping my eyes shut tight to better savour the physical sensations.

Let's be clear, here: this was all a game. It was – to use a cliché phrase – enthusiastically consensual. The fourth wall was flimsier than it sounds when I write it up. Practicality has a way of reining in too ambitious fantasies and that's probably a good thing. If we'd really gone to the woods, I'd have knelt on the hard ground and complained about muscle ache. We'd have had to dodge families having picnics, eager joggers and groups of teenagers trying to start fires. There'd probably be dog shit. In the name of practicality, the guys had to make allowances: they couldn't drive us far in the back of a van with no seatbelts. Nor could they march us – bound and gagged – through suburban London in broad daylight. They couldn't even take us on the short journey without having to pull over and re-input the postcode into the satnav. What's more, in real life even with a deep voice, leather boots and a cultivated air of dominant control, you'll still mutter 'shitting fucksticks' if you misplace the keys to your kidnap den.

Credit to the guys, though, they did their best to maintain a horny atmosphere even when it was clear things weren't going to plan. And even more credit to Simon because, in spite of the fact that there are so many obstacles involved in kidnapping your lovely girlfriend, he bravely leapt over them each and every time, in a valiant attempt to make her knickers wet. When we got to the warehouse I was strung up by the wrists, and whipped from three directions with a selection of implements. I squealed and writhed and clamped my thighs together, desperate for the relief that'd come from a hard, blindfolded fuck. But it wasn't me that mattered: as I gave my best moans and whimpers, Mary got a more intense, more delicious, and consequently more *romantic* version of everything I'd seen from the sidelines. Her cries were louder. Her captors crueller. The red welts she displayed at the end bit more darkly into her pale skin.

And as Simon told her 'Happy Anniversary' and we licked our hard-earned wounds over a glass of champagne, I realised that this was the kind of romance I could really get behind.

You'd never catch me buying a rose bush or scattering petals over a Travelodge duvet. But staged kidnap? Being gagged and pushed into the back of a van so a bunch of guys could pretend to ravish me? It's like my inner pervert wrote the script.

When Did Sex Become The Wrong Way To Show Affection?

(elitedaily.com)

- During a hug -
Him: Ooh, this is different!
Me: What is?
Him: You know – upstairs affection. Usually you only do downstairs affection.

Mark's a fan of cuddles. While that sounds like a euphemism for 'Mark has an unusually large collection of teddy bears that he arranges in amusing tableaux when no one's looking', it's not: he just genuinely loves a good hug. He's pretty much built for cuddling, too: broad shoulders, big arms, an oddly consistent body temperature – like the warmth you feel when you wake up from a satisfying nap. He has a tendency to put babies and cats to sleep as soon as they lie down on his chest. He claims that the cat-sleeping is nothing to do with his temperature and everything to do with how calm he is. That's an affectionate dig at me – I find it tricky to sit still for more than ten minutes without leaping up to check my phone, or the front door, or whether that noise from the boiler means it'll burst into flames and kill us all. Locked in a peaceful hug is Mark's genuinely favourite place to be – never moving or fidgeting or whining that I'm giving him pins and needles. My head on his shoulder, his hand down the back of my jeans, a steadily pulsing erection digging somewhere into my stomach – he could lie like that until the end of time, and he probably would if it weren't for my anxious twitching.

When we first got together, his hugs were a problem for me.

I liked his snogs, for sure – they started soft, wet and teasing before swiftly turning into intense, hard sucks. I have a vivid memory of lying beneath him on an uncomfortable Ikea sofa, wrists pinned behind my head as he smooshed his lips on mine. Slowly. Like he was revelling in the moment when each atom of our lips met, inching closer to the point when he could feel the hardness of my teeth through the flesh. In my head it replays over the course of an hour, and my cunt oozes with wetness before he's even halfway to crushing me. Greedy for the ending, I'd race towards sex like all else was immaterial – whipping up my top and bra, shoving my knickers to the side for ease of access, then letting out a subdued howl of delicious frustration when he'd slow the whole thing down to a languid crawl. His every movement was deliberate, careful and hard. It wasn't lovemaking, like our first mismatched fuck. It was something I'd not had much of before: a different brand of enthusiasm. One that said 'Let's savour this bit right here'. 'This bit' could have been anything: his face pressed hard into my chest, my wet fingertips teasing the end of his dick or the moment when he'd hover, thick cock pressed against the entrance of my cunt, and tell me to beg him for just one stroke.

All that? Top marks. But his hugs could fuck off.

After sex, during that slightly awkward time when you're not sure whether to get dressed or slip under the covers, there are far better things to do than hug. High-five? Sure. Tell a joke? Hell yes. Get off your arse and put the kettle on? Absolutely – with the added bonus that as you slip out to perform your brew-making duties, you get to flash them the bum they've so recently buried their face in.

Mark had a habit, though, of wanting to bathe in the afterglow.

'You're gorgeous,' he'd say, running his hand over my stomach as I tried desperately to suck it in. Moving on, he'd scrutinise every bit of my body that I'd been trained to hate and treat it like it were a brand new treasure he'd unearthed. 'You're hot,' and 'I love your tits,' and 'You've got a pretty cunt,' until I'd grin awkwardly, tensing every single muscle in an effort not to shrink away, eventually giving him the brush-off that he knew was coming:

'Shall we get dressed and go to the pub?'

'I'd rather fuck than cuddle' isn't exactly a confession of wrongdoing – it's certainly better than some of the weirder sexual fetishes I've flirted with – but at the time it felt like a dirty secret. Let's be honest, though: I used to put on *make-up*, and that's not the kind of effort I'd personally go to for a snuggle at the end of the evening. I'd wear high-heeled boots and tiny denim shorts and see-through tops that showed my bra. Sitting on the train on my way to his flat,

I'd plan the evening in my mind: a short walk to his place, ring the buzzer. Watch him run past the kitchen window in a flustered attempt to hide mountains of pizza boxes before I walked in the door. 5...4...3...2... the crackly buzz as the intercom welcomed me up the stairs. He'd usually wear pyjamas. Not to bed: in bed he was always naked. But in the flat, with no one around, he'd slip into a tight T-shirt and loose pyjama bottoms – for ease of access when I arrived at the door. I was dressed like I was off on a date, but my plan was always to skip the 'date' part. All I really wanted was to put together an outfit so suggestive, so easy, so 'fuck me fuck me fuck me' that he'd haul it off the minute I arrived. If I got the timing and the outfit right, I could bypass his desire to take things slowly.

The door would be slightly ajar, and he'd stand a little back from it to watch as I came in. I'd drop my bag, and that was his cue to slam into me, grasping at the bits I'd just dressed so well. Smearing my make-up exactly as I'd hoped he would. Pulling down my shorts and flipping me round, and ordering me to place my palms flat against the wall. There are few physical sensations sexier than cool plaster on my hands, or the waistband of my denim shorts cutting tight into the back of my thighs, as I push my arse out to meet his dick.

It wasn't romantic: it was far better than that. All sweat and slapping and spit-for-lube. Thrusts that made my cunt clench tighter around him to feel every single inch. He'd brace himself against the doorframe to give himself more purchase, and I'd spread my hands for balance and push back twice as hard. Sometimes he'd catch me when my legs started to tremble, placing his big hands just above my hips and physically pulling me up to meet his cock. Other times we'd be too far from the wall, so he'd grab my wrists and use my weight for support: me leaning forward as far as I could, arms stretched out behind me, him yanking on them to keep me upright. We never fell.

This might not be your perfect shag. You may prefer a range of positions – an hour-long session that's more like a workout. You might go for candles and softcore porn, foreplay that feels like a birthday present and lots of lingering eye contact. That's cool. But I'm telling this story so you understand that I don't: I can't. Protracted sex sessions feel more like performance to me than passion and if a guy looks into my eyes while we're shagging I burn hot with a bolt of panic. Does he want me to say something? What face should I make? I think my normal sex face – like that of most people – makes it look like I'm being simultaneously confused, tortured and told I've won the *X-Factor*. Instead of letting him see that and potentially misinterpret it, it was far more fun to turn around and present my arse like a rutting zoo creature, avoiding the risk of eye contact altogether.

What's more, I'm submissive. Not just in a handcuffs-and-spanks way (though I certainly wouldn't say no, Officer), because it feels more all encompassing than that. My submission is a fetish in the traditional sense: I can't get off without an element of that power play. I don't have to be tied up every time, but I do have to feel his hands gripping my waist just a little bit too tight. Hear him call me a 'good girl' when I pull down my knickers. Feel the weight of his body on top of me, and his cock tight inside me, with a crushing urgency that implies I shouldn't escape.

And afterwards, when I'm tingling with filthy pride, remembering the way he grunted as he shot his spunk inside me, I need him to not erase that feeling with a warm and snuggly hug.

When we're done, panting and lying semi-naked on the floor of the hallway, Mark tries to slip his arm under my neck and prick out a line of kisses from my forehead to my collarbone. I make a face.

'Fuck's *wrong* with you?' he asks, like a gentleman.

'I just don't like it.'

'But *I* do.'

'Shouldn't you just roll over and go to sleep or something?'

'It's only 7:30'

So we lie side-by-side, not really touching, Mark growing steadily more bored and aching for skin-to-skin contact. When you first get together, it's natural to avoid letting the other person know that their odd foibles irritate the shit out of you, so it was only later that I learned how excruciating he found this. When I realised, I couldn't understand why he wouldn't be delighted. The idea that he'd be disappointed to not have to follow the list of 'Things Guys Do To Make Girls Happy After Sex' seemed bizarre, as if I'd given him a free pass on doing the dishes, only to have him stare hopefully at the sink and beg for a pair of Marigolds. Now, though, I understand. Let's put aside for the moment his genuine desire to hug, and the fact that when he sees a naked girl, tangled in a post-shag pile in his hallway, his first instinct is to smoosh himself against her. The poor bastard has also repeatedly been told: girls need this. Women will demand at least ten minutes of post-shag snuggle time, during which any heartfelt declarations about how beautiful they are will be very well received. Just as I get angry at the expectation that I'd prefer a lovely hug to a crotch-bumping hallway shag at the start of an evening, he's probably a bit hacked off that he's supposed to 'man up' and swallow affection. That, even after ditching his preferred firm-but-slow style of shagging just to please a girl who wants to hump like the rabbits do, she won't deign to reward him with some warmth.

Imagine: as a woman you've been repeatedly told that guys will always want sex and you won't: disgusting, sticky stuff everywhere, smudging your make-up and dumping spunk-dribbles in the gusset of your knickers. Despite this, you feel a stirring in your pants, have sex anyway and realise that – hey! It's pretty fun! And the spunk washes out eventually anyway! It's a nice revelation, made even nicer by the discovery that men want to do more than just deposit juice into you – they aren't one-dimensional fuck seals, clapping automatically at any hint of a pair of tits. It might surprise us, but we can adjust our expectations and carry on, because if someone wants *more* from you, it's flattering. Contrast this with Mark: he grew up in a world that told him he'd want to shag everything in a two-mile radius, and in exchange for servicing his vital sexual needs, women would make unreasonable demands for affection. He can deal with the sex thing, because it comes as a wild relief that the people he wants to fuck are pretty keen on the whole idea. Me wanting to shag him is a request for more. But if I reject his affection, I'm saying give me *less*. I don't want this. Take all these pesky feelings you have and hide them somewhere I don't have to see.

If it sounds like I'm playing up my emotionless cruelty, it's because I'm used to having to justify any preference I have that might not fit with what Hallmark says on the matter. The 'men like X, women like Y' toss bears as much resemblance to my life as the romance novels that end with 'happy ever after'. Yet every time I say 'I don't like this', someone will pop up to explain that evolution disagrees: I'm supposed to hug after sex because women need to cling to a man so he'll stay and support her babies. Which is interesting, briefly, until I remember that evolution's also given us brains, which allow us to have desires beyond just 'eat/sleep/fuck', and variation, which makes those desires individual. Claire, for instance, is so keen on hugs that she'll even try to tempt *me* into one if I'm feeling pissed and maudlin. Hugs from guys are pretty valuable to her too. She revels in cheesy gifts, enjoys the odd late-night 'miss you' text, and even once – I swear this is true – deliberately encouraged a one-night stand to sleep over at her house. *On a work night*. Claire understands the cookie-cutter love stuff in a way I never will. She wants a man to worship her, and as a result is constantly frustrated when they fail to live up to her exacting expectations. Me? If a guy isn't taking his pants off or getting a round in, I want him to leave me the hell alone. I suspect that makes Claire an easier person to love. While we joke that she's high maintenance because she wants a boyfriend to phone her every now and then, in fact she's far easier to satisfy than I am. A prospective suitor could wander into any branch of WH Smith and pick up a magazine or advice book, and treat it like an A–Z guide – follow the directions, you'll end up in Claire's heart. Conversely, I've got a flashing neon sign pointing straight into my knickers, but you'll get a parking ticket if you stay too long.

It's Mark who loses out here, not me. If he'd kicked me out after the hallway shag I'd have wept once, wanked twice, and wandered on to the next bloke, smugly congratulating myself on not being like everyone else. But Mark's got to take my expectations and his own, and weave them together into something that works. I thought that by pushing away his affection and comfortably embracing his cock, I was challenging the status quo, but I wasn't really. Everything still revolved around what *I* wanted. During those first few months, when we were getting to know each other, he'd tidy his flat before I arrived, make sure he had clean bedsheets, and hope against hope that one night I'd deign to stay over. I never did. Feigning illness, early work, social awkwardness – any excuse I could make to get out of actually sleeping with him – in the snoring sense. Each night he'd cross his fingers as the clock moved closer to midnight, watching me grow limp and relaxed on the sofa and hoping today would be the day I'd say 'fuck it' and hug him to sleep. Then each time his face would fall when I announced, like a budget Cinderella, that it was time for me to fuck off home. I liked that separation, and I was too selfish to consider why he didn't. And sure, wanting him to mop up his jizz with my knickers and give me a high five after sex certainly *sounds* less traditional than asking for roses, but it still ultimately puts him in a place of either delivering what I want or not being worthy. Sucking up his emotions in deference to mine. For the first few months we were together, I congratulated myself on avoiding expectations and dictating a pattern of romance that fit nothing I'd read about in books. Which was shit, of course, because it was still me dictating it.

I didn't stop to think whether Mark would like roses.

Can You Have Sex Without Love & Is It Healthy?

(*yourtango.com*)

Me: I would definitely shag that guy.
Him: That's not special though, is it? It's like if they gave an Oscar to everyone who made a film.

Don't believe the hype about sex with the person you love being the best you'll ever have. It *might* be, and if you're one of those people who believes that 'true love waits' then your married sex will certainly be the best you'll ever get. It'll also be the worst, because it's the *only* sex you'll get, but it's not considered polite to mention that at the hen party.

Let's be honest – first time sex is usually rubbish. You know the other person's body about as well as you know the way to their flat and it can sometimes be awkward to ask for directions. What's more, there are all the typical worries about your body, your technique or the way you shout 'gnnnfh' when you come. You might worry that all your exes have been politely tolerating your foibles, and this new person will be the first to point out that you're doing everything wrong. That you'll be lips-first round a stranger's cock giving it your best tricks and halfway through they'll tap you on the shoulder and say 'have you *never* done this before?' Call me paranoid, but it's a constant worry, ever since a guy stared me straight in the face during what I thought was an extra-special hand job. My ex had taught me this nifty trick and I assumed New Guy's stare was one of profound appreciation, until he opened his mouth and shattered the illusion:

'What the starry-eyed fuck are you doing to my penis?'

Sex with someone you love is different to these one-night-wonders, but controversially I don't think it's the *love* that makes it so. Sure, some people might enjoy it more with chemistry and connection, but like a tedious pedant who insists on explaining how a card trick's done, I'm suspicious of that as the sole explanation. You may well be in love, but you've also had time to learn exactly what your other half likes: a soft, sloppy blow job, a gentle boob massage while you're making out on the sofa, hard smacks across their bum or a cheeky finger inserted at the point of climax. The love explanation sounds great, but I think it's more about familiarity. Understanding the ins and outs of someone's dirty sock basket might kill some of their allure, but it comes hand-in-hand with knowledge of their sexual tastes. For example, I know that Mark often throws dirty socks in with the clean laundry by accident, guaranteeing us both a super-fun surprise when we have to sort it. I also know that he enjoys an occasional five-second full-blown choke halfway through a blow job – where I take it right to the back of my throat until my eyes water and I cough. It's easier to please him because I already know him. But is sex only *ever* going to be awesome if you're in a long-term relationship? If that were the case we could throw the *Joy of Sex* out of the window and replace it with a book that just says 'give it a year or two'. While knowing each other well can mean you're better at pleasing each other, great sex isn't always like a stew that takes ages to perfect. Sometimes it's a massive burger bought for £2 from a fast food shop: quick, easy and intensely satisfying.

I love to live vicariously through Claire's adventures. Last-minute dates on Tuesday night that end with Wednesday-morning hangovers and the lingering smell of lube. Turning down a guy on a Friday only to get bored on a Saturday and end up chatting online, watching him nervously nudge the conversation in the direction of a nude picture or two. These things feel like a heaven I've turned my back on and when Claire talks about it I can't quite work out why I ditched that kind of freedom for hand-ground coffee and pizza on *Game of Thrones* night. Before I met Mark, I dated quite a bit. My week wouldn't be complete unless I'd spent at least two evenings of it on a date with a guy I met on the Internet, and at least one evening where the date culminated in a scramble for the night bus with jizz drying under my bra.

It's not as easy as that makes it sound, though. While I'd love to be able to experience sex in a vacuum (not literally, although shagging in a dual-person spacesuit sounds like all kinds of fun), there are hurdles you have to leap over before you get to go to bed with a stranger. As a woman, my greatest concern is supposed to be the worry that I'm a slut if I shag on the first date. I say 'supposed to be' because we're genuinely getting better at this. Nowadays anyone who carries their own condoms and has a Tinder account understands that a shag doesn't mean a demerit against your immortal soul. In the past, we've had to contend with such nonsense as:

1. If you sleep with him on the first date, you'll never see him again. (He sounds like a tosspot, so it looks like I dodged a bullet!)
2. If you shag him, it's because you want something. (I do! Sex!)
3. If a girl sleeps with one guy, she'll likely sleep with all of them. (Listen: cock is lovely and all, but it isn't heroin. And what's wrong with sleeping with everyone anyway? Oh...)
4. If you sleep with everyone, your hopes of eternal love are dashed forever. Like a piece of sticky tape that loses it's tackiness after a few uses and eventually fails to stick at all. This argument, tape analogy and all, is still genuinely used in some abstinence-only sex education classes. As if women are not only incapable of making our own sexual choices, we're barely distinguishable from stationery.

Women, like men, choose to fuck for a variety of reasons: true love, sheer curiosity, politeness, money, boredom, but often because we're horny and we quite fancy it. We have casual sex for the same reasons guys do; it's just that we have more bullshit to wade through before we can get our pants off. Sometimes from judgemental friends, or newspaper columnists, but tragically often from guys themselves. Patting themselves on the head, they explain that while they'd love to fuck you and know you'd love to fuck *them*, they're chivalrously waiting for date three, because they wouldn't want a lady to feel cheap or easy. Make no mistake that these guys are as annoying as the ones who'll shag you on Monday then never call again. Monday guy may be forgetful, drunk or just plain lazy. Chivalrous guy has decided to hold you to different standards for 'your own good' – it's a special kind of condescension. And it does not preclude them from never calling you again after they've finally fucked you either, meaning you've basically wasted even more of your valuable time on a guy who belongs firmly in the nineteenth century. Please don't date this guy twice: you'll only encourage him.

On top of these, we have the standard problem that any horny suitor faces: rejection. As we fuck for the same reason guys do, so we get rejected for similar reasons too: the person we're chatting up is married, or not interested, or too absorbed in a bloody good book.

Given these obstacles, it's a miracle anyone manages to hook up at all. But humans are resourceful when they're horny, so we do and the excitement and novelty usually makes up for the fact that the sex isn't always skilful. It doesn't take a boring suburban morning to make me miss it – even the most disastrous of Claire's anecdotes gives me a pang of nostalgia as I remember having the freedom of a Friday fuck that wouldn't drag on into Saturday. Claire explains, quite rightly, that it's only really fun if that's what you actually want, and you have no other end goal. If, like her, you want something a bit longer term, then what looks like excitement from the outside can actually be intensely tedious: swiping left through a bunch of guys with three-word profiles on Tinder, schlepping to the other side of London for another doomed date with a management consultant. Worst and most draining of all, those days spent after a particularly great date, and an unusually lovely first shag, waiting for the phone to ring and realising it never will.

I don't want to paint Claire as a loser, by the way: she's the funniest person I know, lively and hot and brilliant. She's the kind of person who arrives at a party (she would not *dream* of cancelling on your party) and provides that mysterious fun catalyst that you didn't realise was missing until she rocked up brimming with it. Yet despite all this she's a dating Sisyphus, pushing a rock up a mountain over and over again, only to watch it roll back down when – three dates in – the guy who seemed quite promising announces he's actually married, or not into her, or votes UKIP or something else appalling. Cruel though we were about the fruit sculptor, at least he was up front about his quirk and saved her having to nod, disarmed, through an evening of chatter about the structural let-down of an overripe melon. But despite the disappointments, she still gets to have that cheap, delicious, fast-food-style sex whenever she fancies it. And although the pre-shag admin might be tedious, having a few conversations about someone's unusual hobby is arguably much simpler than maintaining a full blown relationship: at least you know you can sneak out after shagging without having to go through the rigmarole of 'I'll miss yous!'.

If you want the sex without the commitment, and without all the fumbling that accompanies a first-time shag, then your best option is to pick your hottest, funniest friend and see if you can recruit them to be your fuck buddy. Ignore that stuff about it 'ruining the friendship': a myth often spouted with pursed lips of distaste, as if a pleasurable shag with a friend is something vulgar, like doing a giant fart at a dinner party. It's rooted – I think – in the idea that sex is special and that specialness means it should be a rare treat rather than a regular one. It's just rubbing genitals, though: we're not collaborating on a business venture or co-signing a mortgage. Genitals are fairly intimate things, but it's not like we wear them down through overuse. While your nanna might save her pricey china plates for special occasions, you're a grown-up too, so feel free to use them for fish and chips if you fancy. It's your choice – always. You might not personally want to exchange handshakes for hand jobs with your mates any time soon, but to me the physical intimacy involved in sex is rarely as significant as, say, sharing my godawful teenaged poetry with someone. Unfortunately, not all the guys I've known have agreed, so I've spent a fair amount of time tiptoeing around the significance of sex and detracting from time we could otherwise have spent doing it.

When I was 19, I had a massive crush on my boss. I cannot for the life of me remember why: he treated me with a junior manager's practised disdain, so perhaps I was fantasising to avoid noticing how hellish the work was. If you live in the UK and you own a phone, you've probably received a call telling you to reclaim your mis-sold PPI. I get five calls a day. Drives me up the wall. You may have screamed a colourful range of swear words as you slam the phone down on these people, but have you ever wondered who was responsible for mis-selling all the PPI in the first place? Who cast you into the sales-call Hades from which you cannot escape? It was me. And a team of other phone-hammering students, obviously. My boss stood over me while I did it, encouraging me to screw over a few more people to hit targets before home time. He dominated, like a tyrannical factory foreman, simultaneously flirting with and terrifying me... Come to think of it maybe I *can* remember why I liked him.

One night, over a round of flaming tequilas at the kind of drink-everything-then-burn-the-world party that you can only really appreciate when you utterly loathe your job, I hooked up with him. Outside work, through a hazy veneer of ill-advised spirits, he turned out to be quite sweet and had the kind of shy horniness that I find utterly irresistible. We had a brief hook-up at the party – blow job, snog, smack on the arse (in that order) – and I thought no more about it. The job was just a miserable slog for paychecks before uni beckoned, so it would have taken more than a fumble with the management to keep me there. My boss didn't know that, though, and he clearly wanted to give a stamp of legitimacy to our illicit, secret tryst, so he embarked on a retroactive wooing spree. It was excruciating: nudges and winks, bad jokes and barely credible flirting. 'Morning, Sarah. You look... umm... sexy?' he offered once, with no apparent idea that the rising inflection ruined the compliment. I did my best, but it was obvious that we had nothing in common, bar a horny night at a party and a mutual hatred of the job. Nevertheless, he persisted in asking for dates, with devastatingly tempting lines like 'we should probably at least have a drink together, you know?' so eventually I gave in, and we shared a lacklustre Wetherspoons platter and an hour of painful small talk. There was no lust, or joy: the date was just there to put a semi-respectable stamp on a sordid midnight suck job. Thus, what could have been an excellent sexual memory has been replaced with that of a disappointing evening, followed by an awkward bus ride home as we tried not to explicitly say goodbye.

Compare this to some of the sex I've had with genuine friends, in which all of us recognised the value of sex as a fun thing rather than a hook on which to hang a relationship. Like the night my fuck buddy and I slipped out of the pub, leaving a friend dancing to shit karaoke. We ran round the corner to his flat, let ourselves in and had a frantic, five-minute fuck – the kind you rush through greedily and almost guiltily, like you're sucking down a pint so no one will notice how thirsty you are for it. Or my far-too-short friendship with a couple so beautiful their exhibitionism felt like a public service. They'd fuck and play at swingers' clubs, and occasionally he'd beckon me over with a crooked finger and let me squish my corseted chest against him as he'd press his fingers into the slit of my slick crotch. Afterwards we'd relive the evening's events as we playfully groped each other in the back of a cab.

While I don't miss some of the things Claire has to deal with – all the politics surrounding sex being seen as dramatic and significant, I do miss the people who joined me in playing with it like it was a casual, energetic game. Even if sex with the person you love really *is* the best sex of your life, that doesn't mean other fucks can't be *fun*. Telling people not to shag until they're in love is like telling them not to play tennis until they're in the Wimbledon final. If I'm honest, I kinda miss the qualifying rounds.

7 Must-Have Talks For A Healthy Sex Life

(*mensfitness.com*)

Him: Do I even want to know what that is?
Me: Not sure.
Him: What is it?
Me: A spreadsheet of my best wanking times.
- sigh -

'OK, let's get this over with,' Adam said, sitting down with his coffee and giving me a 'what the fuck have you done *this* time' stare.

Adam: obviously not his real name – his real name is stamped so hard into my heart that using another one gives me a weird twisty feeling in my chest, but needs must. Adam was – if you're keeping count – the eighth person I ever slept with and he stayed in my life for a very long time. He was single-handedly responsible for the vast majority of my 'firsts'. First spanking. First time at a fetish club. First time at a swingers' club. First threesome with a guy. First time I got a sex toy stuck inside me and we thought we'd have to go to A&E. Related: also the first person to fish around in my vagina with a long-handled teaspoon. He was my first utterly compulsive love: I'd simultaneously ache with desire for him and burn with misery because I couldn't believe he'd ever love me back as hard as I needed him to.

It's strange sitting face-to-face in a coffee shop with him, because it's over now and I can't quite comprehend that we're not allowed to touch each other any more. What's more, I have to ask him a pretty awkward question: can I write about you on my sex blog?

One of the most frequently asked sex blog questions (apart from 'do you want to rate my dick lol?') is: what does your other half think? They want to know how the people I write about feel – whether I get their consent and whether there are things I censor because they wouldn't like it. The answer, as with everything, is complicated. You want to be honest about things, and give people a picture of your life that's as true as it can be, given your own flawed memory and intensely biased opinions. But you also want to spare the people you've shagged from the pain of unsolicited critique. The sheer, howling horror of having to relive their sexual mistakes through other people's snarky retweets. It's the 'kiss and tell' conundrum.

When I started the blog, I was sleeping with a few people. A combination of friends, casual fuck buddies (the distinction between 'fuck buddy' and 'friend', while blurry, rests mainly on whether you shag every time you hang out or just when you're both bored and horny) and ex-boyfriends who weren't quite in new relationships yet. I'd also just started seeing

Mark. As a general rule, the more casual the relationship, the easier it was to ask: 'do you mind if I write about your dick on the Internet?' Buddies were more likely to respond with a 'hell yes!' One was so delighted with his eventual write-up that he wore it like a badge of honour on his online dating profile, proudly telling prospective lovers that he'd been given a rave review. Another asked to read what I wrote before I published it. One chipped in some sex advice to accompany the post. Adam gave a far more nuanced answer.

Adam always makes me nervous, because although we've grown apart I have never stopped lusting after him. Worried I might blurt out something weird, I tried to approach it carefully, the way I imagined a mature person would.

'I want to ask you something,' I said, and refrained from adding 'then I want to take you into the toilet out back and sit down hard on your cock'.

'Go ahead,' he said, again with that stare – the dark-eyed, intense look that he used to give me just before he'd grab my wrist and flip me over in bed, pressing his cock up against my arse so I could feel him pulsing against me. My hands shook a little bit and I expect he put it down to nerves. When I'd asked him to meet for coffee he knew this wasn't just a casual catch-up – at the time we were both still raw about our split. He knew I was battling the desire to lean in and suck deeply on the fleshy, warm part of his neck just above the collarbone. The idea of torturing myself like this – by meeting without fucking – meant that no coffee could ever have been casual.

'I want to start a blog,' I said. And before he could get a word in, I reeled off the speech I'd been rehearsing for the last month – about how I really wanted to be a writer, and how they say you should write about your passions and if I'm writing about my passions how can I possibly *not* talk about the filthy things we'd done together? I explained why I wanted to ask his permission – because while any other guy could blur into anonymity, the same couldn't be said of Adam. If I were outed, he'd be too – with the bitter addition that he'd have no control over the stories I'd told.

Before I got even halfway through my speech he stopped me with a sigh and a raised palm.

'Jesus. I *knew* you'd want to do this. I didn't go out with you for so long without realising that at some point you'd want to air all our spunk-stained linen in public.' There's a vague, wobbly smile and for a thudding moment or two I missed him even harder: this guy who had such a fierce grip on who I am.

'So can I?'

He sighed. And he looked at the ceiling for a while, pondering. Turning his coffee cup round in his slender, pale hands. Eventually he lay down the ground rules.

'Do it. Just apply some editorial discretion.'

'In what way?'

'Don't make me a fuck up. Wait. I guess I sort of *am* a fuck up. Please don't make me a *significant* fuck up. I don't want people to read about me and pity me —'

'Shit, of course not!'

'Most writers have one, though. For narrative. The guy who threw away the chance to bang a sex blogger. Or hurt her. Or... you know.'

'Yeah. I know.'

'I'm just saying: don't make me *that* guy.'

For what it's worth, my primary sex writing rule is this: all your stories belong to both of you. It applies whether you're writing a book about your conquests or giggling over your latest one-night stand at the water cooler. Everyone has the right to tell their own stories and unless you consign yourself to a lifetime as a hermit, at some point you will be in one of those stories. That's not to say you should set up a Facebook page and tag anyone you've ever rubbed your bits against: apply that editorial discretion. Just as the right to free speech comes hand-in-hand with the responsibility not to be an abusive arsehole, so the right to discuss your own sex life comes with a big, neon 'don't be a dick' sign: hence the awkward coffee chat with Adam and the subsequent self-flagellation as I try to twist my love for him into insignificance.

When I told Mark about the sex blog, he was far more chilled than Adam. Perhaps because it was early days: we hadn't yet had the kind of sex he'd be nervous to tell his friends about. While he'd have loved the idea of calling me his girlfriend, he knew that'd mean a pretty swift separation without even a goodbye blow job. I was just a girl he liked, who met up with him twice a week or so, then rubbed against him in the hallway of his flat until one or both of us made a come face. We were new, casual and definitely not *significant*. So, as with so much else in life, laid-back Mark made the sex blog chat simple:

'I'm going to write about sex on the Internet. Can I write about what *we* do?'

'Of course. Let's do it again now, though, just so it's fresh in your mind.'

Afterwards, when we were sweaty and knackered and definitely not hugging, he sat up with a jolt, lips twitching like he'd just thought of a killer joke:

'I don't have to actually *read* it, do I?'

Beyond text messages and pizza menus, Mark's not much of a reader. Occasionally he'll stretch to Reddit, but he prefers the posts with pictures. This isn't a way to parade my book snob credentials, it's just a fact: some people prefer pictures to words, and some prefer videos. Or gifs. Why the hell not? A hundred years ago reading was vital to acquire knowledge, but these days you could build an entire house just by watching the right YouTube clips. I only explain it so you understand that reading my blog was, for Mark, a pretty serious commitment. Occasionally he'd swap high-definition porn for thousand-word accounts of our haphazard fucking and give me his feedback via the medium of blow job requests. If a blog was good, he'd point to his crotch, and let me drink in the sight of his prick swelling firmly against the fabric. If it was *really* good he'd put a firm hand on the back of my neck, unzip his flies and nudge me towards him so we could relive the highlight of whatever he was reading.

If you're shy about discussing your own sex life, allow me to try and tempt you to open up a bit: your other half's more likely to confess to their kinky fantasy if you've got the ball rolling with yours. In that way, sexy chat breeds more sex which, in turn, causes more sexy chat: like a virtuous circle in which the hand jobs get more vigorous, imaginative and pleasurable as they're amplified down the chain. Conversely, the less we talk about sex, the less we *hear* about sex from others. No one wants to swap shagging stories with someone who's tight-lipped about their own discretions.

It's like the teenage game 'I have never', which works as an analogy for almost any sexual discussion. If you've never played, then what the hell have you been doing with your life? Grab some friends and a few bottles of the cheapest booze you can find, sit in a circle, and get stuck in. Here's how to play: horny teenager number one states something that they have never done, and those who *have* done it take a sip of their drink. It could be anything – bungee jumping, horse riding, getting an 'A' in a maths test – but, of course, it's never any of those things, because – 15-years-old or not – when it comes to secrets most of us think about fucking. So you start with the simple sex questions:

'I have never had sex in a tent.' (Come on, drink up.)

'I have never had a threesome.' (If you drink here, give a secret smile of nostalgic arousal.)

Then you move on to the more niche activities:

'I have never given head to someone more than ten years older than me.' (Drink and wink at whoever it is across the circle.)

'I have never had to go to hospital to have something removed from my arse.' (Shuffle uncomfortably in your seat.)

'I have never masturbated in a train station.' (Down your drink, please, or I'll feel like you're judging me.)

It's an utterly British way to kick off a sex chat, because while we're often a bit shy about discussing our downstairs activity, we fucking *love* a good drink, so you realise quickly that if you hide too many of your secrets, you'll never get good and trollied. So we say things we've never done, drink to the things we have, then giggle, point, high-five, and cry 'oh my god you *didn't*!'.

No one plays the game itself when they're 30 (we're too busy with fondue and focaccia), but our sex chat still reflects these gleeful teenage rituals. We want to play, because it's fun hearing other people's juicy secrets and you get the excuse to tell people your threesome story without looking like a braggart. So why is it so hard to start that conversation? Because the first person has to set the tone and that's immensely difficult. Begin with 'I have never had sex in the shower' and you might be laughed out of the room – we all did that two years ago and if you haven't you're made to feel like a prude. On the other hand, if you tell people you've never had an orgasm in a swingers' club, you immediately become That Person Who Has Clearly Fucked In A Swingers' Club, and you have to hold your breath while people decide whether to congratulate or condemn you. Most of us want to gauge where we fall on the scale from 'prude' to 'pervert', but those who go first risk the judgement of the next in line. Whether it's envy, disgust, or naïvety about what humans get up to in the bedroom, sexual confessions turn everyone into judgmental tabloid editors.

It's easy to break this cycle, though: talk more. Moral outrage and envy generally spring from a place of ignorance: 'I don't know what that's like, but I have to have feelings about it, so I am either jealous, angry, or both.' If we strip that ignorance away, all that's left is the titillation:

'Really?' someone chips in. 'You've had a wank in a train station?'

'Of course – I paid thirty pence to get into the toilets so I wanted to get my money's worth.'

Cue everyone grumbling about having to pay for toilets and making a mental note next time they have to fork out just to have a piss. Even if no one has done exactly the same, those in the group who may have worried that their solo activities were weird now feel slightly less alone – everyone's a winner (except the people who are waiting in line for a wee). Naturally I don't mean you should wander around your nearest shopping centre with a megaphone. Editorial discretion means not broadcasting your sexploits to people who aren't interested, or at times when they're not appropriate. But in conversation with friends, lovers, ex-lovers and people who follow you on Twitter, don't be scared to talk about your experiences. I promise it's worth it in the long run: you'll get more people horny, hear their stories and advice, and best of all we get to drown out the twats who purse their lips and frown when we do what comes naturally. This, really, is the reason I started the blog. Why I bought a URL, mashed together a few pages, and started writing. When I took a deep breath and set the site to 'live', it was my first move in a very long game of 'I have never...'

The first day it went up, I had 21 visits.

The longer aim, of course, was to get a bigger audience than just a bunch of friends sitting in a circle getting wasted. The second day there were 168 visits, by day four I was up to 500. It wasn't millions yet, but I don't live in a bubble: while my anonymity protects people to a certain extent, Mark isn't naïve, and nor is he miraculously invisible – he knows that one day I may well be outed, and suddenly not only is *my* name out there in public, but his is too. He'll be That Guy Who Fucked That Girl on the Net: thick cock, charming nerdiness and a habit of bracing himself during a corridor fuck that left her trembling and clumsy. When I check these hot things with him, it goes a little something like this:

'You know the other night, when you put the vibrating butt plug in me?'

'I remember it well.'

'And you know how you made that... noise when your cock went in?'

'Uh huh.'

'The gulp, and the sigh, and the way – as you slid into me, rock hard – you had to tense to hold back from coming?'

'Yes, I remember. But please describe it in mo —'

'How you came pretty much straight away, big thick spurts of spunk deep into my cunt?'

'Yes. I remember.'

'Can I write about that?'

'Of course you can. Now get on my cock.'

Mark isn't nervous of being in the spotlight, but understandably when it shines on him, he wants to make sure he looks his best. He isn't a flawless sex god – in a different story he could easily be the guy who didn't spank me exactly how I wanted and had to have it explained to him. Or the guy who mistook my dress for his T-shirt in the dark, and ended up wiping spunk on it. If I were to ignore his request for a positive spotlight I'd be a terrible hypocrite, because I do the same when it comes to me.

One night I came home from a product launch with two free bottles of lube. I don't normally turn up to product launches, because there are PR people there and PR people don't mix well with anonymity. Still, they also often have cocktails and free lube, so I'm sure you understand why I used to occasionally give in, pop on an outfit that doesn't look like I just slept in it and troop off to a launch for some sex toy or other. In this instance it was a lube brand with an unusual gimmick. There were two bottles, with slightly different 'sensory' lubes (one 'tingled' and the other 'zhuzzhed' or something – I'm not an expert, I just smear them on and hope they don't cause a rash). The PR person must have been pretty good, because instead of just asking me to give marks out of ten, she issued me with a challenge.

I turned up at home, half-cut on raspberry daiquiris, banged down both bottles of lube and instructed Mark to take off his trousers. He paused for less than a quantum nanosecond, then whipped off everything below the waist and lay on his back on the bed.

'Do you want to try this?' I held out one of the bottles and he squeezed a bit into his fingers, before rubbing it gently onto the head of his cock. I think he could sense that this was some kind of dare, but he was happy enough to recline, with his hands behind his head, while I took full control. I pulled out a couple of cock sheaths – one tight and black, which fits so snugly round his dick that it's hard to get on without effort, the other softer, more jellyish, which has the kind of sucky texture that he says is reminiscent of a gentle blow job. Cock sheaths make hand jobs more interesting – they're ridged and studded on the inside, the way my own hands could never be, so it's like wanking a guy off with superpowers. I mixed the two lubes, Mark picked a sheath, and we got to work.

Because the sheath was so soft, as I squeezed and rubbed him I could feel his rock-solid dick pushing against the material. Twisting and clamping it round his dick, I could feel the ridge at the head pushing hard against my fingers, and watch the see-through sheath stretch as his cock strained against it.

I love the rhythm of hand jobs. I love the smooth-sticky feeling of lube on my fingers. I like the control – knowing that every kick of Mark's arousal, every grunt and moan, every tingle and twitch is down to me. He put his hands behind his head and looked me directly in the eye. His eyebrows furrowed into a frown as I rubbed faster, squeezed harder. I revelled in the increasing frequency of the slick-slick-slick noises as I rubbed his dick, watching his face grow taut with concentration as he held himself back from thrusting against it.

And then he uttered my favourite three words:

'I'm gonna come.'

Fuck yeah. Oh god yes. Does any three-word phrase have such a beautiful, simple sexiness? Hearing it, ideally uttered with a desperate whimper, makes me instantly wet – eager for the inevitable end, yet prematurely nostalgic for the moment when it's over and I don't hold his climax in the palm of my hand any more. I did what anyone would do and immediately slowed the pace, trying to keep him hanging there for a moment while I took in every detail of his frown, his rapid breathing and the double twitch of his cock just before he came.

Sadly restraint is neither my, nor his, forté. He arched his back, leaning up towards me as he shot spunk into the cup of the sheath. The clear material meant I could see the thick squirts filling it as he moaned. That's what I'd been aching for ever since the PR woman had issued me with the challenge:

'If you can make someone come in less than three minutes,'

she said playfully, 'then you'll know this is a good product.'

If you'd asked Mark what he thought of my sex blogging, he'd probably have mentioned the hotness of reading stories like that and knowing he was the star; the fringe benefit of having someone who comes home with free lube and a filthy idea flashing in her eyes; the opportunity to lie down, pull out your erection and be the test subject for a casual sexual experiment, then dissect the benefits of 'tingling' over 'warming' lube while you drift into exhausted sleep. But he'd also have added the caveat that no matter what the perceived benefits of dating a sex blogger, the fantasy figure people picture from the Internet is only a tiny fraction of the real life fuck-up. You can imagine what it's like to get wanked-off by a horny girl on the net, but it's harder to picture how she'll respond if you eat her last Cadbury's Creme Egg, or sit on the remote control when she's trying to live-tweet *Question Time*. He'd have pointed out the gulf between reality and the write up:

'I bet you won't tell people what you did *after* the hand job,' he'd explain, gesturing at my phone, which displayed a stopwatch app complete with time stamp. I was rubbing frantically at it with a towel and muttering 'shit shit shit shit shit', as I tried to clean off the smears of 'tingling' lube. 'You won't write *that* into the story, will you?'

He'd be right: I didn't. Editorial discretion, see?

10 Simple Ways To Get Laid

(thoughtcatalog.com)

Me: Busy tomorrow – going out with a girl I met on Twitter.
Him: Wow. You made a friend on the Internet who doesn't have an erection.

We live mostly in our own heads, where the other residents tend to agree with us. With the dawning of the Internet, we have the opportunity to surround ourselves with even more people – on Twitter, Facebook, wherever – who have similar views. Barring the odd friend you knew from school who is now suddenly and inexplicably racist, it's rare to read opinions that don't at least partly correlate with your own. When you start a sex blog, it's the same: you're quickly surrounded by others who agree with you and it feels like arriving at a friendly, lefty, sex-loving party. And then more people arrive, and more, until eventually what you write starts to permeate the 'people like me' bubble.

In the first few months, I'd be lucky if I got any comments at all. The odd 'this is hot' and 'do another one about this' would genuinely make my day. Six months in, though, things started to get interesting.

The first phase of this began with the 'I don't believe you' guys. Men who wanted to ask: is this *really* what you think, though? Do you *genuinely* like sex this much? Occasionally they'd throw in a hilarious 'If you believe women want sex, you obviously haven't met my wife'. To which the answers are, respectively: yes, yes, and 'If I were married to someone who belittled me on the Internet, I wouldn't want to fuck him either'. The oddest of this gang were the 'prove it' ones – who'd pop a dick into my email inbox and ask me to demonstrate my sex-positive credentials by hopping on board it.

This usually happened shortly after one of the more extreme blog posts – hardcore BDSM, a fantasy about double penetration, or – given my fairly specific personal tastes – throatfucking. I say 'throatfucking' rather than blow jobs because I mean that very specific thing – the act of tipping my head back over the arm of a sofa so a guy can get his cock right to the back of my throat. It's not for everyone, but it certainly works for me. The sensation of fullness, the horny way he'll grunt to say 'that's right, just there' when he gets all the way in, and the drooling mess it turns me into. When I first met Mark he was wary about pushing it too far – literally. He'd put his hands gently on my head, and thrust tentatively, as if too much force would cause my skull to implode. It was a weird disconnect: the hot sensation of a throatfuck but done with restraint, like someone had spliced a porn soundtrack over a film of a couple snuggling. I'd look up at him with pleading eyes, mentally urging him to make them really water.

When I raised the issue with him (tactfully, I'm sure, like 'why won't you just *go for it*, you wuss?') he explained: 'I don't want to hurt you.'

'But I *want* you to hurt me.'

'What if I hurt you too much? You can't say a safe word with my cock in your mouth.'

'I'll tap out.'

'Like... wrestling?'

'Yeah, like wrestling.'

'You want me to fuck you like we're... umm... wrestling?'

'*God* yes.'

And that was that. A brief, simple conversation, during which he checked what I liked, I told him, and – crucially – he believed me. He didn't go 'wait, but girls don't like this stuff,' or stare in horror at me and gasp 'why would you enjoy something so *degrading*?' He understood that we were having sex, not launching a new political party: the main thing to pursue was grunting, squirming pleasure. From then on, he fucked my face as hard as he liked, safe in the knowledge that I could let him know when I needed a breather. If you're thinking of using the same method, I should warn you that tap-outs work during sex and blow jobs, but you're not allowed to 'tap out' of cleaning the bathroom. I've learned this the hard way.

I realise that not all women like throatfucking – the gagging and the mess and the forceful dominance of it is a specific kink that we don't all share. But what I *can't* comprehend is the number of guys who simultaneously believe that women could never like throatfucking and yet *still really want them to do it*. Pretty please, with a barely-aroused cherry on top. The messages that say 'I don't believe you like this' are annoying, but they're not a patch on the ones who say 'I don't believe you like this, but I want you to do it to me'. Like those people who grinningly insist a particular foodstuff is disgusting, yet still urge you to take a bite. If you're a guy reading this and you're tempted (as many are) to email a sex blogger and say 'Hey, I don't believe you – if you're really a woman and you really like this stuff, come out with me for a drink and I'll throatfuck you in an alleyway,' I'd strongly urge you to reconsider. If you begin with the premise that the other person couldn't get any pleasure out of sex, you'll turn it into a self-fulfilling prophecy. What's more, while it might sound great in your head, 'prove it' almost never works as a chat-up line. Other things that don't work as chat-up lines, but which have all popped neatly into my inbox to thoroughly ruin a Thursday morning include:

'I've fucked quite a lot of women but they were all frigid. Can I fuck *you*?' I've paraphrased slightly, because no one's ever *this* up-front about it, but 'my exes were awful – how *you* doin'?' is a surprisingly popular technique.

'I don't like online dating, can't talk to people in person, have already tried to fuck all my friends, and I'm not willing to pay for it. So how do I get laid?' Paraphrased again, but you'd be surprised how many dudes ask me for 'advice' on sex problems, simultaneously eliminating any potential advice I could offer. What they're looking for, really, is for me to descend from on high like a sex angel, land neatly upon their penis, then milk them to an easy climax.

While annoying, these offers are like champagne and free cake when compared to some of the scarier ones, so brace yourselves or skip to the next chapter if this kind of stuff creeps you out.

In the last couple of years we've heard a lot about rape and death threats on the Internet. As a general rule if you're loud, outspoken and female, you'll have a bunch of people who want to punish you for one or all of these things. I'm lucky enough to be white, straight, and cisgender (i.e. not trans – my gender matches the one I was assigned at birth when the midwife cooed 'ooh, a girl!'), but if you don't also tick these boxes (and others besides) then it could be even worse. Top-shelf pricks with nothing better to do will set up 7,000 Twitter accounts from which to hurl abuse. I've been lucky – *more* than lucky, from what I can see of other people's comments – that I've rarely had this kind of shit. The people who take a strong dislike to me are rarely angry – just disappointed. They're guys who arrive for the sex, drool excitedly over their keyboard, then splurge their outrage when they discover I'm a feminist. 'I thought better of you!' they cry, hurling toys out of the pram. 'I'm taking my erection elsewhere!' It's not exactly terrifying. The worst I'll get from enemies is the odd 'you're a slag lol', and my own mother could do worse than that.

But that doesn't mean I'm immune from that creeping trickle of terror when an anonymous stranger gets in touch. The scariest thing I get comes not from enemies, but fans; not rape threats but rape *promises*. Moving away from paraphrases, these are direct quotes:

'Bitch, you need to come to [City] so I can facefuck you.'

'I was wondering whether you fancied meeting up so we

can push your limits a bit? How hard do you think you could take it from me? Vomiting's a given... have you ever vomited blood?'

The second one in particular – what am I supposed to do with this? I opted for 'going to bed for an hour, shaking in terror and praying that this guy would never find out where I live'. When I'd recovered, I emailed him to explain that vomiting blood was generally considered a bad thing and that mentioning it – in your very first contact with someone you might want to fuck – is, to put it mildly, a bit of a turn-off. Save that for your fantasy play, with blood capsules from the pound shop around Halloween and do it a very long time after your first ever date. He meant no harm: his second email was apologetic and lovely, and I suspect if he'd known how genuinely scared I was, it would have been even more so. But there are plenty more where he came from: men who don't understand the maze that women have to navigate when they're fulfilling their sexual fantasies. The guy who told me he wanted to act out a blog post I'd written about fucking a stranger in an alleyway – I just needed to let him know where I'd be and he'd come and fuck me without ever learning my name. The one who invited me to – of all things – a wedding, and said that if I'd be his date he'd do whatever I liked in the hotel afterwards. No matter how hot an idea, a stranger eagerly offering to fulfil it is going to set off alarm bells, because women usually have to consider their safety as well as their sexual whims – we'll get to this later.

The emails aren't all depressing, though: occasionally I'm tempted to reply to the 'prove it' guys with quotes from some of the women who email to say 'I'm into that too, thank you for writing about it!' Or 'Can we have some more posts about piss-play? I'm trying to show my boyfriend why he might like to do it with me'. One couple sent a joint email to explain that they took turns reading my stuff to each other on long car journeys, entertaining each other with passages about furtive masturbation, while trying to avoid indulging in the same and causing accidents. It's harder to talk about praise, because I am British and alongside heavy drinking and apologising for non-existent faux pas, one of my keenest hobbies is self-deprecation. Still, it's worth mentioning the praise because even though quoting people who've said I'm good is about as comfortable as tearing out my own fingernails, it makes it feel like my horny ramblings are worthwhile. No amount of rape 'promises' could counteract the joy of these virtual high fives. That moment of affinity is awesome – the 'me too' that makes you feel that little bit less alone.

Alongside bad emails and lovely ones, I've saved the largest category for last: dick pics. Large, small, flaccid, erect: if you have a fetish for contextless, blurry phalluses then the Internet is the place for you. To this day, I have no idea what the attraction is in sending your cock to a total stranger, but I have to put my hand up and accept a large chunk of the blame for the sheer quantity I received. When I launched the blog, I enjoyed looking at dick pics, so it seemed reasonably harmless to let people know, on my 'contact' page, that if they needed a box to stick 'em in then my inbox was open. 'What the hell?' I thought, foolishly. 'I like a good penis, surely I'll enjoy a few dozen of them? And perhaps it'll stop people sending them to ex-girlfriends, or other bloggers who've asked them not to.' How wrong

I was. Here's a rough timeline of what happens when you solicit dick pics:

Oh, that's a lovely cock.

Another.

Oh, this guy wants me to rate him.

I'll just repl-

And this guy.

I'll just email them to say than—

Ten more cocks arrive.

I'll just say 'ta' then and...

Jesus, *more* of them.

And, oh, another.

Wait, that's the guy from ten minutes ago again!

How do I...?

First guys email again to ask what I thought of their cocks.

Ten more cocks arrive.

If you'd asked me four years ago if I thought it was possible to get thoroughly sick of cock pictures, I'd have laughed you out of the room before looking at some pictures and settling down for a lovely wank. Now, though, I am well versed in what it feels like to be utterly drowning in cock and I can tell you it ain't as awesome as I thought. It's as if, upon expressing your desire for cake, you were offered not just a slice or two but a whole patisserie and the previously friendly baker insisted on shoving piece after piece into your mouth. You try to smile through the cake overload but he just shoves in more, shouting, 'You LOVE cake, don't you? Go on then, eat it! Then rate it out of ten! TELL ME HOW MUCH YOU LOVE MY CAKE!'

Around this time, Mark and I had our first major argument. Like all good arguments, it started with a close-cropped iPhone snapshot of a dick. He wasn't pissed off that I spent my days sifting through other people's cocks, no: delighted to be exploring his filthy side, he thought it might be fun to send a picture of his own. I can't blame him for assuming that I'd be quite keen – like I say, I initially enjoyed them and his is a pretty top notch example. Let's get that out of the way, because we're seven chapters in and I haven't yet waxed lyrical about it. It's thick, straight, perfectly proportioned and as photogenic as they get without Instagram filters. I can hold it in my palm and squeeze down hard on the solid girth of it, wrapping my fingers around and revelling in its satisfying weight. Length-wise, about average depending on what you count as average: when I sit down on it I feel comfortably full. Stretched taut and satisfied, not so much it hurts. In short, if I could draw my perfect cock (and like most people, the best I can stretch to is a comedy 'spunking cock and balls' line drawing) then I'd have produced something very much like the appendage with which Mark pokes me awake first thing in the morning. So I wasn't annoyed because he sent a picture, I was annoyed because he sent it *anonymously*. His email – mentally filed under 'yet another fucking dick pic' – languished unopened for well over a week, as if his actual penis wanted to make a point about me being unable to see the wood for the... other wood. To me it was just another missive from another horny stranger, whose knob would sit patiently while I got on with my day-to-day life, ready to be picked up when I had time to peruse the new entries.

When he told me he'd sent it, I was bizarrely angry, and it took me a while to figure out that it was because it felt like a test. As if he wanted me to prove my affection for him by picking his knob out in an identity parade. But he forgot the key point: anonymous genitals are rarely hotter than the genitals of someone you actually like. No matter how great his cock picture, I'd have loved it more if he'd simply attached a name to it.

I was used to anonymous guys on the Internet saying they wished they knew me better (translation: could fuck me whenever they wanted), so the idea of Mark wanting to swap places with them was baffling.

'No one wants to be the *anonymous guy* on the Internet!'

'I thought it'd be fun!'

'But... you guarantee a fuck whenever you pick up the phone to me!'

'I know. I just thought you might reply!'

'Brace yourself for this, Mark, but anonymous guys on the Internet... *really want to be you*!'

'I know. There's no need to be a prick about it. I just... I thought you'd recognise me.'

Now that I've calmed down and stopped popping blood vessels over it, I can see why he might have been upset. If your penis is the physical asset of which you're most proud, not to mention the one which your lover has most frequently got misty-eyed over, perhaps it's reasonable to conclude that she'd be able to differentiate it from the others. But when you're a sex blogger, it's not that simple.

'Would you recognise my cunt in a line-up?'

'Of course.'

'A line-up with over *five hundred* other cunts?'

'Do... do you really get that many?'

No, not really: I rounded down.

In the first two years I was blogging, I received 708

pictures and videos of people's penises. Not from 708 individuals – there were 395 *people* in total who sent me a snapshot; it's just that some people chose to send far more than one. The gentleman who sent no less than 12, to show every single angle, in every possible state, currently holds the record for the most photographed knob in my inbox. Some guys included lovely emails: 'I enjoyed your blog so much I thought I'd return the favour', or stories in which they imagined banging me in a variety of interesting ways. Others included items they'd found lying around their house – for scale, you understand. Tape measures, TV remotes, a bottle of Mountain Dew: all acceptable cock accessories to the gent who wants you to get a realistic picture of what he's packing. I know it's tempting to read this and go 'Christ, what an awful world we live in', but my general reaction is quite the opposite: isn't it amazing that, on request, total strangers are willing to show you their private parts and expect nothing but a rating in return?

I've never actually rated the cocks, despite the strange and insistent requests of cock owners that I give them some kind of review. Partly because I'm not sure what to give them – marks out of ten? A grade drawn in red pen with accompanying smiley or sad face? Mainly because, if what you're after is a carefully considered view on whether your penis is up to scratch, I'm the last person who can give an unbiased review: it's like asking an alcoholic to recommend you a decent wine. If I were to rate your dick, I couldn't possibly guarantee that my score would be representative. I'm a fan of variety, so you'd get bonus points for unusual stuff (I'm looking at you, guy who masturbated while wearing a nappy). I'm biased towards video, especially if it includes all the gorgeous grunting noises you make when you're straining for orgasm. I'd probably give you a higher rating if your hand was gripped tight around it, showing the throbbing redness of a really aching cock head at the moment just before you come. If you include jizz: ditto. If the picture includes your face (and precious few of them do – the last thing you want is to send something and have someone reply with 'Barry? Oh my god I recognise you from school!') then you'll get a better rating just because I can see your eyes and imagine them narrowing slightly as I whisper dirty words into your ear. Some people would get bonus points for making me laugh (like the guy who apologised that his wank video had *Alien versus Predator* playing in the background), and others would get marked down for sending pictures even after I'd asked them to stop. As I did – as I *had to* – eventually. I realised that scrolling through schlong after schlong just so I could check my email was getting me down. Rather perfectly encapsulating the mantra 'be careful what you wish for', something I used to love had become no more than admin: a blossoming guilt about having to reply to everyone, and a gnawing misery that the dick pics I used to like had now become a weird static background noise to my life. I changed my email address and added a message to my blog asking people to please stop sending them. Two years later, they almost have.

As a rule, the ones that still trickle through are from people who genuinely worry. Is my dick too small? Is it weird-looking? The 64-million-dollar question: am I *normal*? If you have genuine questions about your penis, I urge you not to send it unsolicited to a sex blogger (or anyone, come to that). Feel free to visit the Wikipedia page on dick, which is incredibly detailed, and examine the average sizes from around the world. If you care about shape, appearance or any of those things, you're better off asking your real-life partners – or in some cases your GP. I can think of no situation in which an anonymous person on the Internet will have a more useful dick-based opinion than the people you're actually sleeping with. If I'm never going to sit on it, hold it, or put it near my mouth, my opinion on your penis is essentially irrelevant. I mean I could rate the new line of Louis Vuitton handbags if I wanted, but I'm never going to buy one, so why should Louis give a fuck?

The same is true, to a certain extent, when people ask me for sex advice – another of the common things that falls into my inbox. 'Will my girlfriend like X?' people ask, or 'Should I tell my partner that I'm into Y?' I'm the worst possible judge of your sexual proclivities, because I can never be objective. I have a vested interest in getting people to talk about sex, and I'm actively aroused by your unusual fetish. Given that, who am I to tell you whether it's 'weird' that you wank over pictures of people scrubbing the toilet? So fascinated am I by people's unusual fetishes, I regularly spend hours falling down the fascinating hole of Google search terms – even more fun than an inbox trawl, if you ask me. It takes a while to build up blog traffic, but once you're at a certain level (after six months to a year or so), if you log into your traffic stats you can see lots of terms people have searched for which eventually led them to your blog. Alongside the obvious ('dirty sex stories', 'sex blog', 'girl hard fuck love'), you get a whole heap of more intriguing ones. '3.8 inch cock picture' was deliciously specific, and

'Halo 4 blowjob' gave me the sexy shivers. Ditto '12 boys fucking', although it made me wonder: does the fantasy require that *specific* number of boys? If one was too ill to make it to the gang bang, or brought a friend, thus turning it into an odd number, would the sexy dream be ruined? The questions people ask in searches can be as enlightening or depressing as the comments. I hope, for instance, that the person who asked 'Can girls enjoy anal?' landed on a page that gave a suitable 'Hell yes'. And I *really* hope that the person who asked 'what if a girl's vagina is fucked 50 times' now understands that the vagina isn't a limited-use item, like a sponge that gets gnarly after two weeks next to the sink.

By far my favourite terms, though, are the ones which open a shiny new window into sexual options I'd never considered. Amidst the '6 girls get gang-banged' and '50 shades of fisting', there's an occasional flash of a sexual dream that I feel deserves a bit more treatment. One person, and I imagine them searching hopefully for an erotic story that reflects exactly the nuance of their fantasy, opened up a new browser tab in search of:

'My wife fucking a butternut squash.'

Not just any vegetable: a butternut squash. And not just any woman: his wife. The best thing about running a sex blog is this window into people's dreams and fantasies – as with 'I have never' and other sexy chat, it's one of the nicest ways to explore the 'am I normal?' question, and get an answer you didn't ever expect. You might prefer looking at cat gifs or cute baby pictures on Facebook, but this is where I get *my* warm and fuzzy feelings. We live in a world in which one person's ultimate bucket list item involves a quick trip to the local supermarket, and a loving connection with the woman he married. I don't know about you, but I hope one day they sat down together with a bottle of wine and a delicious winter vegetable risotto and he swallowed the courage to have that conversation.

Work-Love Balance: 8 Tips On Juggling A Career And Couplehood

(femalenetwork.com)

Me: Thing is, it's easier to ask for a fuck than to tell someone great that you love them.
Him: For you. Easier for YOU.

Let's jump forward by about a year. The blog's getting around 15,000 visits each month now and actually counting them is nudging 'obsession' rather than 'hobby'. Given that the sex blog is starting to take over my life, it's a miracle I haven't been fired yet. Why not? The simple answer is: no one at work knows. The more complicated answer is that I run myself ragged trying to make sure they never find out.

The closest I came to that terrifying confrontation happened shortly after a tedious meeting. A colleague and I had left the room and I'd launched into a hissed mini-rant about how – as ever – two guys who knew slim-to-fuck-all about what we were supposed to be doing had utterly dominated the conversation. The old trope that no one will listen to a woman's suggestion until a man repeats it? Sadly true, in my experience. Perhaps not in *every* meeting, but enough that I've been frequently tempted to include a Powerpoint slide telling specific individuals to STFU. The rant obviously sparked something in her mind, because she turned to me and said, 'Hey, there's this feminist blog you should totally read, I think it'd be right up your street.'

'Ooh, that sounds good,' I said, while simultaneously trying to prevent myself nervously vomiting into the nearest recycling bin. All I could think was 'Christ, I really hope it's not mine.' That sounds arrogant – the chances of my blog being known among my colleagues was probably fairly low. But I've been paranoid since I started it, and no matter how unlikely it is that your plane will crash, if most of your waking thoughts involve plane crashes, you're bound to over-egg the odds of it actually happening. What's more, it'd be odd to assume that my colleagues are any less interested in sex than the rest of us. Naturally, as a colleague, I only see this woman's professional face: even during moments of frustration, she remains so composed you wouldn't suspect she's secretly planning to push a senior manager down the lift shaft. But after 5pm I've no idea – for all I know she runs a sex blog herself, and has her own deluge of dick pics to deal with.

I've never told any colleagues about my blog. While I'm at Company X – renamed to avoid potential kerfuffle, not because I genuinely work for an organisation that sounds like a Bond villain's cover story – I have to avoid any crossover between my Net life and my day job. It sounds hypocritical: 'We shouldn't be ashamed of sex!' isn't a particularly credible battle cry when it comes from the mouth of an anonymous person. But there are quite a few things that get in the way of me putting my real name out there along with my blog. Email 'promises' are a significant one; employment is another.

I maintain a completely separate, unremarkable online identity: a Twitter and Facebook account under my real name, where I'll have the kind of conversations you'd expect from a late-20s office worker. 'Great cocktails this evening!' 'Sign this petition!' – a sycophantic parody of the uncontentious aspects of my life. At the same time, I tweet and write as *Girl on the Net*, a persona I carefully curate to make sure that very few of these identifiable (read: boring) details sneak in – holidays, real-life friends, complaints to South West Trains about late-running services, that kind of thing. It means that each event in my life has to be chopped in two, packaged and presented in two different ways.

For example, on a typical Sunday morning I'll get up, curse my hangover, drink coffee and eat toast. Then I'll slip back into bed, where Mark's still sleeping. I'll strip off from the waist down and slide neatly into the space created by his curved body, then wiggle my arse against him until he wakes himself up with morning horn. When he rolls on his back to stretch, he'll use one big hand to pull my body on top of him, position my face perfectly still in front of his as he teases the entrance to my cunt with the head of his dick.

'Horny?'

'Yeah. Awake?'

'Fuck yeah. Sit on it.'

He half-yawns, then stifles it with a sharp grunt as I slide right down to the base. For a while he lets me fuck him vigorously, grinding in just the right way until my legs go weak and I come – cunt gripping tight around his cock as I bury my face in the sweaty morning-smell of his neck. When I'm spent he grabs my hips with both hands, holding me firmly while he fucks into me from beneath. If I stay perfectly still, clenching all of my muscles like I want to squeeze the orgasm out of him, I know that when he comes he'll call me a good girl, and in half an hour we can do it again.

On Twitter, under my real life name, that looks a bit like this: 'Having a lovely #LazySunday – never getting out of bed!'

As 'Girl on the Net'? 'One hangover, two fucks, three coffees: #SundayWin.'

See what I mean? In 'real life' I go to work, pop to the pub and make crap cheesy puns to pass the time. Over on the blog, I write long essays about period horn, or strap-on sex, and other things that don't usually make it past my brain filters and out of my mouth. Few companies have explicit policies about what you can and can't say about period horn, but – like all large organisations – Company X believes the way its staff behave in private can damage its reputation. It's not that your sex life should reflect the brand values ('We need to embrace openness and blue-sky thinking, so let's hold this meeting naked in a field.'), it's more about damage control. You may never be told explicitly – 'no online chatter about religion, politics, or dick' – but if you're working full time you'll likely have a contract clause about not 'bringing the company into disrepute'. These clauses are all well and good when they're preventing people from making racist statements in a press release, or punching a client at the Christmas party, but 'disrepute' is a nebulous and ever-changing thing. Back in the 1980s, no company would ever expect its employees to tow the company line when they'd clocked off – we'd have been a weird society in which the only people who could speak about politics or sex were unemployed. But social media now means that your opinions aren't confined to chats in the pub: they're available to anyone who wants to look at them and woe betide you if they aren't on message. In my working life (not just at Company X) I've seen people disciplined for anything from talking about their charity work to saying something that conflicts with a company policy long ago forgotten. People who run personal blogs have been asked politely to take them down: they're critical, you see, of a certain government department, and we do occasionally ask that department for funding. If your company works with consumer brands, you might be asked to refrain from criticising their services, or that one time you were sold a sandwich that turned out to have a pube in. If you're outspoken about your sex life, you'll probably be asked to either tone it down or shut it down. Increasingly, people are being asked to sign away their right to an opinion in exchange for an employment contract.

So what do you do? Well, if you'd rather not shut up – and if there's one thing that's true of me it's that I'd *rather not* shut up – then you'll need to go anonymous. Not just 'user264' anonymous, you need to build a whole new online life. First you must invent a new persona – let's call her 'Sarah', although obviously that's not your real name – from which to set up the rest of your profiles. Sarah's your sex blogger and she has no friends at all. Why is she such a loner? Because it's data that matters here, not companionship: you might have any number of super-trustworthy friends, but Facebook will never be one of them. For example: remember all those guys who sent dick pics? If you sign up to Facebook under a real name, you might start getting told to make 'friends' with them. And vice versa. By the way, you may think someone could never know your real name if you email them an anonymous cock shot from 'KingOfBantz@hotmail.com', but if you've used the same email for Facebook then whoever got your knob gets your profile picture too. So, always use a separate email address – one you never use for actually emailing. Do the same with Twitter, Snapchat, Instagram, all the rest. Never, ever join LinkedIn. To be honest, that's a pretty solid rule no matter what you blog about: LinkedIn was created by the devil to work out who'd give him the cheapest price for their soul.

Alongside your spare profiles, ideally you get a spare phone: every app you use to manage your online life wants one thing from you – more data. That means you'll get popups every now and then prompting you to 'merge your contacts'. Hitting 'yes' means the app will out you as a sex blogger to everyone in your address book. Your parents, friends, ex-shags and colleagues: they'll all get told to follow SexBlog, and receive a tiny, avatar-sized picture of your tits into the bargain.

There are loads more hurdles to jump: when journalists contact you, give them a fake name. Choose a few fake names so that if your real one gets out it only adds to the confusion. Log in on different browsers. Password-protect the shit out of everything. Pay cash for your phone top-ups (like *The Wire*! Only much, much shitter!). Tweeting on the train? Stop. Someone's reading over your shoulder. Get a friend to pretend to be you at social events. Ideally, a few friends: ask them to tap their noses when asked for their Twitter name, or say 'Oh, I'm "Girl on the Net" but I don't like to talk about it.' You need to become like a cross between an enthusiastic spy and a cold-hearted, friendless hermit. It's not that your friends aren't trustworthy – there'll be some people you trust to know your double identity. But friends get drunk and let things slip and they're all on Facebook too – block them. They're the people most likely to give away your secret except, of course, for yourself.

No precaution can guarantee your anonymity – one day you might leave your phone unlocked and a colleague happens to glance across as a tweet pings through: '@ girlonthenet I just read your blog about butt plugs!' Perhaps an enthusiastic reader probes your close friends for details, and after a few beers they accidentally refer to you by your name. Maybe you attend a sex writers' convention, under a pseudonym, prevent anyone finding out your real name, then as you're patting yourself on the back on the way back to the train station, realise you left your wallet in the pub. Clubcard, drivers' license, real name and photo and all.

Alternatively, one day you're coming out of a meeting, having a hissed feminist rant to a colleague, and she turns round and recommends a 'great blog':

'I think it'd be right up your street,' she told me, and my heart started pounding so loudly I could have sworn she could hear it. I put on what I thought was my best 'neutrally interested' face. Please please please don't let it be m—

'It's called "Girl on the Net".'

Fuck. I couldn't pause to think: what would I do in a normal situation, where I didn't have all these anonymity rules ticking constantly around in my head? So I asked her to repeat the blog name. I wrote it down, with a kind of earnest and deliberate precision as if I've never heard the name before – I looked like a child learning to write the word 'hello' for the first time. I'm surprised she didn't lean over and help me with my handwriting.

If you're reading this and you're the boss of a large company, or even a small one: please do us a favour and cut this shit out. Whether you like it or not your staff will have lives outside work. There might be legitimate no-nos – if someone says something so awful in their personal life that you think it'll affect how they work, then that's a different story. If you run a bar and your bartender makes a homophobic comment on Facebook, chances are there's a bunch of your customers who aren't getting the kind of respectful service that they should. But if they're writing blog posts about strap-on sex, and your company neither makes, nor has any official opinion on strap-ons, then any damage to your brand is only a reflection of the knee-jerk emotions of bigots. And in these gloriously politically-correct (read: polite and sympathetic) times, pandering to bigots is the most brand-damaging thing you could do.

Given all this worry, you'd be forgiven for imagining that I do something desperately important over at Company X HQ, but I don't. For some reason 'what do you do for a living?' is a pretty frequently asked question on my blog. Until now my answer's always been a dismissive 'I work for MI5' or 'Maybe I'm *your* boss'. The reality is less fun and

I don't even jazz it up by wearing stockings and suspenders underneath my suit to the office, like some kind of secret sex superhero. I do web stuff: online writing, managing websites, writing social media policies; checking a bunch of graphs to see if they've gone up or down; training people to use Twitter; training people *not* to use Twitter if they're one of the aforementioned opinionated types. Occasionally I get to chair meetings, and while my Powerpoint sucks, I always have the best meeting biscuits. Company X (just like, I imagine, whoever *you* work for) doesn't appreciate me or my meeting biscuits, but they definitely pay the bills. Which is useful because I have a mortgage and I occasionally like to buy sexy black ankle boots, or invite hot guys to theme parks to finger me on the rollercoasters. I try not to mention that last bit in the office, though: I'm great at this professionalism thing.

As well as hiding my sex stuff from my 'real life' persona, the separation is tricky the other way round too. At this point, my blog lags a few months behind reality, as I try to fudge timelines as well as names to keep the guys I shag anonymous. As I got closer to Mark, this time-shift led to some pretty odd moments. I'd be dolling myself up for an evening with him, then publishing posts about getting whipped by a casual fuck buddy: a guy who'd long since departed for someone less flaky than me. I'd revel in reminiscing and forget whom I was actually supposed to be seeing. Picturing this blast from the past turned me on – he was a quiet, calm, dominant who wore leather gloves sometimes, and used to whisper orders to me while we sat in public restaurants. With just a short sentence or two he could send my heart straight down to my knickers so I could feel the pulse running through my crotch.

'Do you want dessert?' A raised eyebrow at the end of the meal. He knew the answer was 'no'.

'No, I don't want dessert – I want you to take me home and then beat me until I weep.'

So, generously, he did.

He'd position me face-down on the bed, buried deep into the pillows so I couldn't see what was coming. Flip my skirt up and tug my knickers down so they rested at the top of my thighs – framing my arse to give him a canvas to paint red with pain. I heard him behind me, picking up various things, and I couldn't guess what they were until he smacked them hard down onto me.

Whack.

A slipper. Six strokes. Hard. The sting from the previous stroke barely finished before the next one would begin. When I bit down on the pillow and cried out, he'd give me a rest, and I could hear the slow slither of his belt being pulled through the loops of his trousers. The swish as he looped it round his hand. The crack as he tested it's flexibility.

I wriggled and pushed my arse up to greet it as he swung it hard down onto me. I love the belt.

People reading the blog probably thought that was a recent thing – in fact the story had been sitting in my drafts (or my head) for a good six months before I published it. It went live long after the welts on my arse had faded, just as I was falling hard for Mark. The other guys had started to disappear as I realised with intense frustration that this soft, shy, intensely nerdy guy was starting to creep into all of my thoughts. Like patient Rory from *Doctor Who*, who waited (with the help of some timey wimey stuff) for a thousand years for his errant, excitable girlfriend: when I started to realise how great he was, Mark was still there waiting. Even during mini-panic attacks about whether I accidentally tweeted a blog link from the work account, I'd get bursts of warmth spreading through my chest, gleefully anticipating the next time I'd see him, fantasising about exactly what he'd do. Probably not the belt – it's not his thing as much as mine – but hopefully a deliciously snuggly over-the-knee spanking, with my knickers pulled down to my thighs and his big hands alternating between smacking my arse and dipping roughly into my cunt.

As more of the stories started to focus on him, I made a worrying realisation: Mark and I were monogamous. A six-month delay in what I was publishing and the separation between blog life and real life had lulled me into partly believing the myth of the horny sex blogger – that my life was still the cycle of eat, sleep, fuck, repeat that it had been over a year ago. It had distracted me enough that I failed to notice the c-word that had been hovering ever since I first met Mark: rather stealthily, we'd become a couple. Not a *couple* 'couple' – we didn't go shopping in Ikea, or host dinner parties, or masturbate secretly when the other was out, quickly closing browser tabs to hide our personal fantasies. In fact often, when I had a wank, I'd think about him. He'd embraced the dirtier things that made me tick ('OK, so you want me to fuck you like the people in the porn I like?') and come up with a few things that I'd never thought would make me so shivery: bending me over the foot of the bed and belting my thighs to the posts, strapping me open so he could fuck me so hard that my hips bruised purple on the bed frame. Pinning me down while I squirmed with delight, lubed-up cock teasing the entrance of my arse, for agonisingly long minutes as he bit my neck and called me a good girl. It was a far cry from the quick, playful fucks I'd had with others and I started getting greedy for it. Sex and Mark became synonymous, until time spent with someone else felt like a waste of what I could otherwise be spending with him.

It wasn't just the sex, while I'd have loved to pretend it was. With Mark, I felt more like me than I had with anyone else. It's hard to explain, but here goes: when I do the washing up, I sing. It makes the chores less painful, and it means that for ten minutes or so, I can flush out the bit of my brain that won't usually shut up: the bit that tells me I have a million things to do and that I shouldn't be wasting time on show tunes. Sometimes I can hit the high notes, and sometimes I wail off-key. The quality of the singing is not important: it's about the fun.

When Mark opens the kitchen door and pops in to put the kettle on, he does something which goes against all of his immediate gut instincts at the time: he *doesn't tell me to stop singing*. No 'cut it out' gestures, raised eyebrows or putting his fingers in his ears. He doesn't sing along, or tell me I'm good enough to go on *X-Factor* (I'd be one of the people they feature in the 'you're having a laugh' section early on in the show), but he smiles – not just tolerating my fun, but actively loving it. As with singing, so with everything else. Syrupy e-cards encourage us to 'dance like no one's watching', but I think what's even better is to find someone who'll watch and smile, no matter how shit you are at the Macarena. Mark embraces all of my qualities, even if they're annoying or tricky or un-photogenic. The way I snore and talk in my sleep, the panicked way I run through the station to make sure we're ten minutes early for a train, the way I come home late at night and fling my shoes across the room before lying face-down on the carpet. In front of other guys I'd suck my stomach in to try to look sexy, laugh at their crap jokes or pretend to be cool for a fuck. It took a while to put my finger on what Mark did that was different: he never made me stop wanting to sing.

While I was stalling on the whole 'couple' thing, scrabbling for dates that didn't feel like a shadow of my evenings with Mark, he made a pretty wise move. He had a quick fuck with someone else – the only one since he'd met me – and the gut-punch of jealousy made me re-think my desire to shag other guys at all. If I want him this much, why am I pretending that I don't? Why do I write about him with the same casual nonchalance that I write about number 30, or number 12, or whichever other lover I'm reminiscing about this week? I could still remember and write about the people who'd come before, but Mark commanded my attention in a way that others didn't. No matter how much I loved variety, I couldn't deny that I also loved Mark.

If the sex blog is supposed to be honest, I might as well go the whole hog. A six-month delay is one thing, but holding back emotion from blog posts about Mark felt like telling only one side of the story. So I set out to write something so mushy, so loving, and so utterly vomit-worthy that it would surprise even romance-loving Mark. Ridiculously, I was more terrified of posting something cheesy than any of the other stuff – the belt and the boss blow job and the kidnap fantasy. When I realised just how important he'd become, I tried to suppress the kick of rage – angry at myself for letting him become too good to lose. It's not exactly surprising, but it made me realise that I have far too many of my own prejudices about love: that it's somehow more about Ikea-shopping and dinner parties than lust. That it's a pathetic shadow of the freedom I had when I wasn't tied by emotions to Mark. So when I published something on the blog that praised his character as well as his cock, I was terrified that it meant the end of something. Not sex necessarily, but certainly independence: I'd spent so long mastering the art of being happy on my own that having actual feelings for a guy seemed like the worst kind of failure.

To which Mark, inevitably, replied: 'Fuck off, dickhead – it's lovely.'

He'd been waiting for me to say something. Patiently, while I raged and wrote and reminisced about past fucks, Mark had been sitting quietly on the sidelines hoping that one day I'd have an emotion that was more articulate and loving than just 'please please *please* let me sit on it'. So when I eventually wrote something that fell firmly into the 'romance' category he didn't run away or get hostile or awkward and uncomfortable: he emailed me to tell me he'd read it, and that it was lovely. That he had stood outside work smoking a roll-up, browsing my latest posts, and as he came to the part about him he shed a tear or two of happiness.

It didn't feel, like I thought it would, as if I was giving something away. It felt more like I was inviting him in. After all, he had become part of something now – this odd, secret, anonymous world. When one of his colleagues popped out for a smoke, and asked him: 'What are you reading?' he got another step further into my life. He got to experience that heart-thumping panic combined with the illicit thrill of a shared secret.

He got the chance to say: 'It's nothing,' knowing it was anything but.

Why Relationship Drama Is Addictive, And What To Do About It

(*hookingupsmart.com*)

Him – gesturing to a very messy flat – All of this is brilliant.
Me: What's brilliant?
Him: Life.

If you asked Mark to write you a romantic comedy, it'd go a little something like this:

Boy meets girl. They share a pizza. They fuck.

If you wanted more than ten minutes of material, he'd ask you – with genuine confusion and concern – why on earth the boy and girl couldn't keep doing that for the duration of the film. Pizza's nice, fucking's nice – what's not to love about the chance to do it over and over?

Every year on his birthday, Mark does the same thing: he meets up with a couple of friends, they go to the same restaurant as last year, eat the same meal and head home at the end of the evening. After watching this ritual the first year I knew him, I asked in the second if he'd like to do something special.

'I'll pay – I've saved some cash. Is there anywhere you'd like to go, or anything you'd like to do?'

'Nope. Same place.'

'We can do that on your actual birthday, but would you like to do something extra? Dirty weekend, go-karting, one of those red-letter days where we drive tanks or some shit. Theme park?'

'You know you don't need to be on a rollercoaster to get fingered, right?'

Scowl.

'But... it's your birthday! Don't you want to do something *special*?'

'Yep. I want to do the special thing I do every birthday.'

Here's Mark's theory: your birthday is supposed to be the one day each year where you get to do whatever you want. You invite the people you like, pick a place you enjoy, and go there to enjoy it. So if you decide, on your birthday, to do something drastically different to what you'd do on an average day, then you're not having one special day – you're having one failure of a life for the other 364 days of the year. I'm not entirely sure I agree, but it's hard to argue when he pins me down on the sofa and pushes his face into the crook of my neck.

Slipping a hand casually down the back of my jeans, fingers spread, like he wants to grab as much of me as possible, making me squirm against him, he asks:

'Don't you want to do *this* every day?'

Maybe.

Often in rom-coms sex is the climax of a long, drawn-out courtship. The 'yes!' moment when two people realise they're in love, and tumble into bed together having finally realised that it's their destiny. In real life, it's far more likely to happen the other way around: you shag someone for long enough and then realise that they've grown on you. This sequence makes for shit entertainment, though. There needs to be a will they/won't they drama to keep people guessing, not just a gradual shift towards that moment when one of them grabs the other's arse and says 'want to keep doing this?'

The first time Mark told me he loved me, I cried and tried to leave, sensing a trap. Like a tediously melodramatic teenager, I couldn't quite cope with his plodding, secure, quiet conviction that if we were having fun we should just keep on having it. My own custom romance script would include a bit more excitement – an explosive fight scene against secret agents, maybe a car chase or two. A kidnap. Definitely extra characters. Lovely though Mark's story is, something in me hankers for a bit more plot. When he says 'Let's keep doing this', there's an answering voice in the back of my mind that tells me life can never ever be that easy. I think what it means, perhaps, is that life can't be *fun* if it's easy.

It's like they say: you need the dark to appreciate the light. Adam and I were one of those dark/light couples. Only instead of light we had weird, sticky, fetishy sex and instead of darkness we had simmering rows and desperate, sobbing despair. We'd got together when we were at university, a ripe age for developing odd baggage and gathering grudges which could be nurtured and sharpened ready to wield at a later date. Also the perfect time for exploring the most interesting fantasies that bubble up from your teenage mind.

Our relationship had a shitload of plot: in the space of an hour we'd snap from sweaty, urgent sex in the toilets of a pub to drunken, tearful arguments by the bar. A row about our weekend away was smoothed over as soon as the car door slammed, replaced by joking and flirting. Adam trying to concentrate on the road, gulping down his arousal as I gently squeezed the end of his dick through tight jeans.

'Keep your eyes on the road.'

'*You* keep your hands in your lap, woman.'

I'd squish my legs together and sit on my fingers to try and keep myself from touching him, then get weird flashes of sadness when he'd forget to suggest we pull over. By the time we reached our destination the cycle of arousal and rejection had me wound so tightly that a single look from him could have me thudding with joy or cringing inside with misery. In case it isn't clear, this was mostly my fault (he's not 'that guy' – never 'that guy'). While both of us had a tendency to navel gaze, our most passionate fights were kicked off by my pathetic insecurity.

One night we dressed up and drove, with much of the aforementioned dick-touching, to a friend's house for a spanking party, and this story could have ended so much better if I'd kept my mouth resolutely shut.

The party was a fairly regular thing: once every few months a couple we knew would host a dinner, and we'd turn up squeezed into corsets, latex, or whatever took our fancy. I'm cheap, so I cheerfully reused the same corset umpteen times and my fishnets were so ragged they were basically glorified string. It didn't matter, though, the point of the party wasn't to impress: I was there to drink, chat, and bend over the nearest heavy object so one or more people could flog me till I squealed. I liked the parties because I got to meet new men. Adam came along because I liked to meet new men, and – to my intense irritation – he wouldn't be pressed further on the other aspect. With a jealous girlfriend and a roomful of semi-naked friends, Adam was understandably reluctant to have the 'do you fancy her more than me?' conversation. It's almost as if my constantly pressing him to confess that he looked at other girls' arses was a *teeny* bit of a mood killer.

While I was mingling, and not-so-subtly hinting to dominant older men that perhaps I'd been a really naughty girl, Adam caught the eye of their female equivalent - a beautiful domme. She was tall, broad and angular: perfect eyebrows, cheekbones, pouty red lips. Everything about her was neat – from her hourglass body in latex to her short, painted fingernails. She looked like she'd stepped out of a comic book: Dominatrix Woman, transformed after being bitten by a sadistic and horny spider. What's more, she was utterly lovely into the bargain. Her appearance said 'back off' but her smile said 'bloody lovely to meet you, shall I put the kettle on?'

When she spoke to me she caught me a bit off-guard:

'Is that tall, skinny one your boyfriend?'

'Umm... yeah. Pale? Scruffy hair?'

'Yep. Do you mind if I play with him?'

If I were a dog, this'd be the moment my handler would place their palm on my neck and croon, 'Easy girl. Eeeeeasy.' But I swallowed it. After all, Adam was hanging onto her every word, and she looked excited to get her hands on him. More importantly, what kind of terrible, hypocritical twat would I be if I'd lifted my skirt for any guy who looked vaguely interested, then banned Adam from getting a beating of his own?

She took him into the play room, where a huge frame had been erected in the middle of the room. He stripped, lowered his eyes, whimpered, and said 'please' as she whispered gentle commands. She touched him all over, lingering on his hipbones, and the soft dip beneath them that I used to love to kiss. She pulled out whips, lay them reverently on the bench nearby, before selecting her favourite and lashing hard strokes into his naked back. I realised halfway through that I'd been holding my breath, and I think he had been too. Mine was partly relief that she'd invited me in to watch - that I got to be a part of whatever hot stuff was going to go down. His, I suspect, was pure lust – a combination of submission, exhibitionism, and the knowledge that for the next half-hour or so he needed to do nothing but endure and obey. He was rigid in position: his cock pressed firmly against the bench in the middle of the frame, his wrists cuffed to the top bar. There was nothing for him to do but close his eyes, bite his lip, and make those choked moans in the back of his throat that he made when he was trying not to come. She squeezed his arse and called him a good boy, and she snapped on latex gloves and held her hand over his mouth. And all the time I watched: horny and happy and squirming in my seat. Imagining the moment when we'd get home and I could strip him naked again. Kissing each bruise and welt and blurry red hand print. Later in the party I did my usual rounds – batting my eyelashes at various older guys and getting them to whip down my knickers for a quick over-the-knee spanking. And I enjoyed it even more knowing that the red marks on my bum would match those on Adam's: that we could compare later as we relived the hotness of the evening.

I'm telling you this story because it was as close as things came to perfect: a fun night together, a filthy hot scene, that delicious feeling when you know that someone else wants your partner too, and when sharing their arousal makes you feel even closer. However it's also an excellent example of what frequently went wrong. There was a delicious fuzzy feeling afterwards, when I poured her a glass of cheap Cava and we compared compliments on his marks, but that feeling disappeared as soon as we left.

I willed myself so hard not to say it. The night had been amazing: Adam had been amazing. Superdomme had been amazing. We'd made new friends and new memories, and I could still feel the tingle of other guys' hands on my bum, warming me even as the car seat froze my thighs. 'Don't say it,' I reminded myself sternly. 'You don't need to.' But my ridiculous, insecure, pathetic brain whispered the question over and over until it seemed more important than anything else. Like a truthful answer to this would either make or break me forever:

'You fancy her more than me, don't you?'

God, those words are so *small*. I hate them, and I hate myself for asking this question yet again. Because as I remember the night in its fullness – as I remember *every single night* – Adam's happiness is always shadowed by that question.

Do you fancy her more than me?

Each time I asked I'd despise myself more, and get more frustrated by his answer. There were only so many times he could say 'no', and only so many ways to say 'I love you'. Only so many times I could pick over and over our relationship, looking for a crack to fix, before I realised I'd worn the damn thing down to dust.

Still, it's passionate, isn't it? Dramatic. Say what you like about Adam and I, but at least we had fucking *plot*.

'I agree, mate. Love's boring. Let's move to Thailand.' So says my best mate, let's call him Dave. Everybody's got a mate called Dave, right? Well, my Dave is everybody's mate. He'd kill me if I called him a hippy, but that's essentially what he is. He grins his way from party to party, gathering new friends and acquaintances like a nice top gathers cat hair. I once left him waiting outside a train station while I ran to top up my Oyster card. Gone less than three minutes, I returned to find him singing 'Bohemian Rhapsody' with a homeless guy and passing him the details of a newly opened squat.

Dave slops cider over the table as he puts the drinks down. There are four pints for two of us, because the pub is crowded and life's too short to queue. 'I don't have any money or anything, but if we went to Thailand and freelanced, we could earn enough to buy a bar or something and just, you know, have fun.'

'Except we won't because we're grown-ups now.' We all have our role to play, and mine is the killjoy.

'*Fuck* being grown-ups. The good thing about being a grown up is that you get to decide when you want to *stop* being one,' Dave says.

'Are you coming to this rave later? It's in an abandoned school. You might meet someone dramatic there.'

He knows it's a 'no' before I even have to say it: I've never been a clubbing person. When I was 16 I did what all 16-year-olds do, and sneaked into clubs that were lax about their door policy. I detested them, yet was convinced by my friends that clubbing was a universal joy: everyone must like it, or why would people queue for so long to get in? So I tested other ones – indie clubs, rock clubs, cheese clubs – anything with music I knew the words to. Each and every time I'd reach midnight, have a vague claustrophobic panic attack on the dance floor, then sneak out and hail a taxi home. At this point in the story I'm pushing 30, which joyously means I don't have to pretend any more: I hate nightclubs. They're rubbish, overpriced, hot and boring. And sure, clubbing might be more fun if you're on drugs, but so is housework. Drugs make boring things fun: that's why they're popular. If you'd rather sit in a quiet pub, having a chat and a pint and a pasty, then please come and join *my* club. We have plenty of peanuts, and we never miss the last train.

I suspect that Dave sometimes uses me as an excuse to slow down. When he needs a break from partying, he calls me, and I show him how dull life can be by telling him that my only news is that Mark killed a cake I was baking.

'Killed?'

'It's a sourdough. Like you have to let it live for a while and feed it before you turn it...'

'Wow. You're... baking? This is dangerous.'

'You don't even care about my cake, do you?'

'No. Next question.'

Like me, Dave is a cynical bastard, and suspicious of

anything resembling commitment, so he acts as Devil's advocate, and helps me pour out my ridiculous fears about Mark:

'I'm going to die one day. And what if I die and I've spent 20 years just pottering along with Mark, doing all the things that are just "fun"?'

'I can literally *hear* the scare quotes you put around fun,' he points out.

'They *are* fun. Incredibly fun. Like the other day, we walked round all the shops in his area, buying up all the different types of Coke...'

'Riot.'

'Wait, I haven't finished. We had, like, Cherry Coke and normal Coke and Diet Coke and Coke in a glass bottle and Pepsi...'

'Then you chucked them all away and did something less dull?'

'No, we...' He's looking at me like I'm weird, and I realise too late that this is a 'had to be there' story. '...we did a taste test.'

'With Coke.'

'Yeah.'

'Fun.' He rolls his eyes, but he's smiling, because he kind of understands.

'So that was fun. But then we also do things that are really...'

'Grown up?' And as he says it I realise that 'grown up' sounds like 'finished' – it's the phase that comes after the happy ever after, like 'settling down' and those other things that imply a well-earned rest. But surely you can't have a happy ever after if there's been no drama on the way. If

I'm going to reach a finish line, I want to be damn sure I'm sweaty before I break the tape.

'I just don't want to regret being with Mark, and missing out on all the other stuff.'

'Look,' he explains, and when it comes out of his mouth it seems so obvious. 'You could regret being with Mark or not being with Mark, but you won't know that until you split up. You just need, in the meantime, to realise that you can have fun without doing grown-up things you don't want to do. Like marriage and that. You think marriage is claustrophobic and horrible, like clubbing, whereas Mark thinks it sounds like fun.'

He's right. Mark talks with a sickening ease about the future – he's as keen on commitment as I am on independence, and the casual confidence with which he discusses children, moving in together, joint bank accounts, has certainly not been lost on Dave. He ticks them off on his fingers one by one:

'Marriage? No point in it. Joint bank accounts? Very bad idea. Babies? Same thing but with a bit of extra vomit. OK, they're cute and you can customise them to a certain extent, but that's a minor difference.' I can't work out if by 'customise' he means 'dress them up' or 'teach them to do your bidding' but either way, he's right, right?

'But if I don't want any of this stuff, then why am I in a relationship? What if, when you're in love, you just *do* have to do this? What if everyone else is right?'

He looks around the beer garden – young couples mingle with older couples, groups of friends giggle at the start of a Big Night Out, and we sit somewhere in the middle, with a pint in each hand and a brimming ashtray between us.

'Nah,' he says, with reassuring confidence. 'I reckon we've got it about right.'

'Are we boring?' I ask Mark a few weeks later, as he rolls a cigarette on the sofa beside me. We're making an effort not to watch TV, because the night before I made a comment about how much TV we watched, and he's either making a sarcastic point or being lovingly sensitive to my whims – I can't work out which.

'No. We're not boring,' Mark says, matter-of-factly. He lists off some of the stuff we've done recently and he's much better at remembering interesting things than I am. I remember stuff like box sets and blow jobs – like me kneeling on the floor and sucking his cock while he completes a battle on Halo 4, challenging myself to make him come before his in-game character gets shot.

Mark remembers things like the time we went on a London 'zombie run', and got painfully high on adrenalin. Naturally, as a pair of total nerds, we'd already had in-depth conversations about what we'd do if Z-Day came and the human race turned into a pack of brains-hungry zombies. So while other participants giggled and ran from the paid stooges in crap make-up, Mark and I set up rescue missions to save people trapped in stairwells and tricked a group of rude teenagers into providing cannon fodder while we helped the rest of our team escape. He points to our third or fourth date at London Zoo, where one of us made a joke so funny we were in hysterics for half an hour: neither of us can remember the joke, but the fact that we can remember the laughter is – as he quite rightly points out – evidence of fun somewhere down the line. He reminds me that once, when I was away for a week, he found a top and some jeans that I'd left at his flat. Naturally, he dressed a cuddly teddy bear up in them, arranging it neatly on his bed in vaguely human form before texting me a picture and a cute 'I miss you' message. Adorable text sent, he settled down in front of the telly and proceeded to get incredibly stoned. So stoned, in fact, that when he went into his bedroom later on and was confronted by the ghastly teddy-bear-girlfriend hybrid, he says he screamed so loudly it woke the neighbours' baby.

'See? We're not boring,' he declares, putting the finishing touches to his cigarette and laying it to one side for later. As if to prove just how rock and roll we are, his eyes light up with enthusiasm and he screams: 'Fucking hell! We've got *crumpets*!'

Living the dream, I tell you.

I put the kettle on and he makes crumpets and we sit in his living room staring at the walls, wondering what it is two late-20s party types should be doing on this special day. Oh – did I mention it was New Year's Eve? That's important. To stay in of a Saturday and eat crumpets is forgivable, but to do the same on New Year's Eve is a crime against youth. We should have been freezing on the south bank of the Thames in anticipation of a midnight firework show, or at a house party where our friends smoked weed and looked askance at the twitchy stranger who always turns up to sell cocaine. At the very least, we should have had the decency to fork out £20 for a ticket to our local pub. We'd be deafened by a shit covers band, but at least we'd maintain our dignity.

But we didn't. Instead, we polished off a packet of crumpets, sat on his living room carpet, and sorted his small-change jar into neat piles of pounds and pennies. You know, that pot of coins that you keep persuading yourself you'll cash in but you never do, because you figure sorting it isn't worth the meagre £15.26 you'll get at the end? But lacking anything else to do that evening Mark and I thought it'd be worth tackling. We sat down, dumped the coins on the floor, and made a start. And it was bloody good fun. This tedious task became intensely enjoyable, simply because he was doing it with me – chatting, making jokes, fighting over the only visible five-pence piece that we both wanted so we could make a neat pound out of silver change. I'm telling you, we counted the *shit* out of those pennies.

Perhaps it took me so long to realise I was in love with Mark because his version of love was so different to what I expected: we never had 'the chat', in which we agreed to call each other 'boyfriend' and 'girlfriend', or had awkward formal meetings with each other's family. Mark slips into everything casually, taking his theory of 'if it's fun, I'll do it' to every single aspect of his life. I was fun, we had fun, end of story. I kicked against it because it felt like there should be a 'moment' – something dramatic. That relationships should be based on one specific decision, or at least an argument in the rain that ends with a healthy bout of make-up sex. But there were very few of those moments with Mark: just an ever-so-gradual descent into coupledom. Sofa sex, pizza, box sets, jokes, and eventually a cosy New Year's Eve in which we sat together on his living room floor counting the pennies from his small-change jar. As we bickered and fought over who'd get the last five pence, it reminded me of my mum and stepdad turning pages at the piano and Lucy's husband holding shelves while she marked out the drill holes.

It's a crap storyline for a dramatic rom-com, but maybe love is exactly as everyday as this. Anyone can swoon over champagne at sunset, but how often do those big, sparkly things happen? Once a year maybe? It's easy to be overwhelmed with emotion during an intimate anniversary dinner, but over the course of a whole lifetime with someone we'll spend far more time doing the dishes together, or waiting for the kettle to boil? Neither Mark nor I can promise an eternity of pleasure or a happy ever after: all we can guarantee is that we'll spend a lot of time together. In that time we'll have adventures and joy, of course, but we'll also have to do everything else: sweeping leaves from the garden, looking up train times to go and visit his parents, arranging standing orders for the gas bill, washing up, watching telly. Love isn't always dramatic or emotional: love is menial and everyday.

Perhaps, for Mark and I, it's about counting pennies.

How To Seduce Each Zodiac Sign

(*huffingtonpost.com*)

Him: Where shall we go next? A pub where the beers are cheaper, or home, where we don't have to wear pants?

Sometimes people ask me how they should go about getting laid. What are the best chat-up lines, how do you seduce someone, and how can you be so goddamn sexy that people just won't resist leaping into bed with you immediately?

To say I'm the wrong person to ask is a dramatic understatement.

My seduction style combines incompetence with desperation to create a heady mix of awkwardness. I am direct and to the point, but not in the commanding way that you'd expect from, say, an Internet sex kitten – more like what you'd expect from an extra-terrestrial who has been told the bare minimum about sex, but wishes to engage in it for research. In my house, whispered seduction is less common than a shout of 'Sex time!'

I'd love to say that this is born of familiarity – that Mark and I are simply comfortable enough together that we feel able to ask for sex without having to jump through scented-candles-and-lingerie hoops. But I don't think it grew from anywhere: it has always been that way. Tearing my clothes off in the hallway was his traditional technique in the early days and that still works if we're feeling particularly passionate. But equally successful is his tactic of approaching me after he's stepped out of the shower, grabbing my hand, and sliding it inside the towel so I can feel how hard his dick is. My equivalent is more verbal, but no more skilled: I'll lie on the bed in my knickers, stick my arse in the air and say 'Fuck me'. If I'm feeling particularly coquettish I might give it a rising intonation, as if I'm asking if we have any ice-cream left for dessert.

The beauty of this kind of seduction is that it isn't overworked, and it doesn't require a huge amount of confidence. 'Fancy a shag?' is a delightfully easy chat-up line, because you're not putting much out there beyond the fact that you *do* fancy a shag, so if the other person chooses to decline (as we each do occasionally – sometimes there are important things to read on Reddit or valuations to hear on *Storage Wars*), it's not the end of the world. The idea of doing more than simply *asking* for a shag has always seemed a bit counterproductive to me – why on earth would I bother persuading someone if they weren't already tempted?

Hence the first time I talked Mark into bed went a little something like this:

'Do you like chips? There's a great chippy near my house.'

'Sure. Let's go.'

Brief break for an awkward bus journey, chip purchasing and stilted discussion over chips in my living room. After we'd eaten, I gathered up the greasy paper and wandered into the kitchen. Mark sauntered after me, and as I turned round from the bin, he was a bit closer than I'd expected him to be, so I leaned in for a slightly clumsy kiss.

Mark: 'Oh. Nice.'

Me: 'Shall we go to the bedroom now?'

Mark: 'Sure.'

I'm not saying he's *easy* as such, but apparently he'd only followed me to grab a Coke.

Equally successful seductions have begun with such witty lines as 'have you ever had sex in a tent?' and 'what would you do if I sucked your dick right now?' While this no-nonsense seduction style works well for me, it does leave me feeling like a bit of a fraud when people get in touch via the blog looking for tips. 'How do I get laid?' they ask, as if I'm some kind of sex guru. When I fumble and stutter and say 'Um, well, you just sort of find people you like, talk to them for a bit, then ask them to have sex with you' I feel like a total let-down and I suspect they feel pretty ripped off too. Maybe that's why shit seduction guides like *The Rules* and *The Game* have such dedicated followings: they talk as if there really is a formula, even though there isn't. While a doctor can tell you that if you want to stay healthy you need to eat your greens and get regular exercise, charlatans still make millions with detoxes and juice cleanses and 'this one weird trick'. Deep down we all know it's bollocks, but we still desperately want there to be a secret.

Here's a secret that's not-so-secret: I know fuck-all about how to get anyone else laid. That doesn't mean I won't try to help, of course. Giving advice is fun because it makes the giver feel like they're doing good without having to solve problems directly, like donating money or volunteering to run a marathon. It also makes us feel wise, despite the fact that most of us would never follow our own advice. I rarely feel wiser than when I'm telling other people the right thing to do – and I certainly feel better handing out tips than I ever feel when I'm failing to live by them.

When I began the blog, I wrote a series of posts titled 'What is not wrong with you'. Every time I spotted a new instance of people feeling shit about a particular aspect of their body or behaviour, it went in the 'not wrong' bank. Over the course of the first two years, I told people that there was nothing wrong with being a tall girl (or a short guy), nothing wrong with being fat, nothing wrong with being ginger, having bodily functions, or refusing to shave your bikini line. 'Fuck society!' I exclaimed, through my Internet megaphone. 'Love your body as it is! Don't let judgemental people tell you how to live your life!' It's all true, of course: if people are shitty to you because you have ginger hair then they are weapons-grade arseholes who deserve nothing but contempt. If people treat your body (too fat, too skinny, too muscular, not muscular enough) as some kind of moral barometer by which they can assess your worth as a person, then these people, likewise, are cunts. Unfortunately it's easier said than done – while I stand on Mount Internet hurling commandments down to any poor fucker who'll listen, I'm not always practising what I preach. I suspect the same is true of almost anyone who gives advice: we're not saying 'Be like me, I'm perfect', we're saying 'Don't be like me, I'm *rubbish*'.

A couple of years ago Mark and I went to a nudist beach. It's exactly the kind of thing you'd expect a confident, horny sex blogger to do. Being naked! Yay! Seeing naked guys! Double-yay! Surely, you'd think, I'd be sashaying excitedly onto the sand before whipping off my towel for some skinny-dipping and the chance to get Mark to rub sun cream on my tits. Except it wasn't like that at all – Mark was the one who was keen to go naked. He's always enjoyed nudity – it just feels good on his skin. The faded pyjamas that he wears around the house are apparently so stifling that even those get yanked down every now and then to get some air on his too confined junk. Being naked is natural, fun and freeing, he told me, and it'd be nice if we could do something *he* enjoys on holiday, rather than sticking to my personal routine of traipsing round museums then getting smashed on cheap sangria. So I packed up my appallingly inadequate body, and we drove down to the local nudist beach.

This is the point at which I have to describe myself and it's not going to be easy. You know how some people are so terrified of spiders that, if there is one in the room, they have to keep their eyes fixed firmly upon it so they know where it is at all times? I am one of those people and have the same fears about my body. I hate so many things about it, to such a ferocious degree, that I know it in direct and obsessive detail. On a basic level, I'm very tall, broad shouldered, a size 14, 16 or 18 depending on how recently we had Christmas. I have dark-ish hair depending on how recently hair dye was on sale in Superdrug. And I wear glasses and have a couple of piercings and all the things you'd expect a pervy nerd to sport on their face. That's just the basics, though: what other people would see. Imagine my body, as I do, mapped out in sections. Each section, roughly an inch square, contains a new and unspeakable horror. This bit has a bright red stretchmark. This bit has those weird red chicken-skin spots that appear on my arms for no apparent reason. This bit is too fat, but not fat in a curvy, pours-nicely-into-latex way, fat that gives me an odd shape: dodgy hip dips that look like I'm wearing too tight knickers. Don't get me started on body hair, either: if bikini lines, armpits and legs were my only body-hair worry, I'd be happier than I've ever known.

But I should be confident, right? I said so myself on the Internet. The world's scorn, and society's request that women present in just this way at all times, means nothing when compared to my freedom. I should march onto the nudist beach with a middle finger and a 'fuck you' to anyone who'd tell me I shouldn't be there. I know I should. But the problem is, it's not as easy as that. Your rational mind says 'I don't need to hate my body just because it doesn't meet impossible beauty standards', but your emotions lag way behind. After all, if it were that easy to throw off centuries of conditioning about the right 'beach body' then the ideal of a 'beach body' wouldn't be dangerous: it'd just be a question of replacing our cultural wallpaper with more diverse models, then giving ourselves a pat on the back. In reality, we have to do lots more, including struggling with our own internalised body hate even as we loudly condemn the idea that any body should be the target of hatred. It's an odd kind of narcissism – *your* body's fine and perfect, but *my* body is so howlingly grotesque that no amount of triumphant rhetoric could justify me showing it naked in public.

What I'm saying is that when we arrived on the beach and stripped naked, I didn't stride around confidently, or gleefully embrace Mark's love of the wind on his naked butt: I spent 15 minutes sobbing face down into a beach towel and wishing I could fall off the planet.

It's natural, of course: any persona we present on the Internet is always going to be an edited version of our real life self. Scratch any story that seems cool on the Net and you'll find a fuck-up lurking beneath. Some of my sexy stories (Mark cuffing my legs to a spreader bar and holding me steady while he fucks me) cut off before the failed conclusion (a cramp just after he's come that leaves me howling 'argh, shit, ouch, bollocks' while he scrabbles with keys to try and whip the cuffs off). When I write a porn story about what I want Mark to do to me when I get home (pushing me to my knees and wrapping a belt round my throat) I don't subsequently write about what *actually* happened (I walk through the door and burst into tears because the taxi driver was mean to me on the journey).

It's the easiest thing in the world to be a 'sexpert', if by 'sexpert' you mean 'someone who'll answer your questions about sex with an air of arrogant authority'. If what you want, however, is someone who genuinely knows what the hell they're talking about, I'm going to utterly disappoint you. There are some great people out there who have qualifications and years of experience in sex science, therapy or any of the other things that mean they've a genuine leg to stand on when doling out advice. I'm not one of them.

What's more, there are plenty of 'sexperts' who have nothing even vaguely approaching expertise – they've a handful of experiences and a giant bag of assumptions, and they mix and match these things to try and offer us a secret 'formula'. Top Ten Ways To Blow His Mind In Bed, or Body Language Tricks To Get Her Panting – all that bollocks.

When people disagree with me in blog comments, I'm usually quite pleased: I can either hone my arguments, change my mind or realise that it was worth writing something in the first place. The comments that hurt, though, are these ones:

'Who the hell are you to give me sex advice?' or 'what could you possibly know?'

They hurt because they're right. I'm no one. Just because I love a particular sexy thing, it's no guarantee that someone else will. That's why I so rarely give practical advice: 'touch him here' or 'whisper these words' or 'try this position'. I'm not a peddler of cheap sex tricks, just an incompetent girl chasing pleasure for herself, but when people ask questions it's easy to fall into the trap of pretending I've got the answers. Am I, in urging people to 'love their body' and 'use this toy' and 'tell your fantasies to your other half', starting to sound like the self-appointed sexperts that I so frequently get frustrated with? Really, like most of us, I'm just making this stuff up as I go along.

Inevitably, when you muddle through with things, you end up being wrong some of the time, and I still cringe when I remember some of my earlier blog posts. I used to make thoughtless pronouncements about the Way Things Should Be, such as 'everyone basically likes spanking – it just depends how hard they want you to do it!' Shudder. I was making reference, really, to the idea that spanking's just another form of touch, and even if you're not the kind of person to go to a party and request that guys with erections beat you till you tremble, you may still enjoy a quick gentle smack during the throes of vanilla-flavoured passion. But, of course, that was wrong – spanking is like drinking tea: not everyone likes it, and if you claim everyone does then some people will end up doing it just to be polite. If this stuff had stayed in my head where it belonged rather than being spewed forth onto the Internet, I wouldn't be aching with shame as I write about it now, but thanks to the blog all my weirdly shitty old opinions are still online for anyone to access. Like that time I told people they didn't need a safe word if they were doing BDSM, and ended up looking like I was making a case for 'no means maybe'. Not just awkward, actively dangerous, as so many people pointed out to me at the time. I wasn't saying 'no means maybe', of course, it was far more banal than that: I was just annoyed at the idea that if you want to have the kind of struggling, dark, role play that I enjoy sometimes with Mark, you don't need to establish 'Purple dinosaur!' as your specific escape route, you just need an escape route that works for both of you. Personally, Mark and I have never had a safe word, because it's pretty clear between the two of us when it's time to call it quits. It's the difference between me saying 'no, please' in a sultry voice and me saying 'ow fuck, bollocks' in the voice I use when he's left the kitchen light on.

It's easy to believe that people on the Internet never change their minds and there's definitely a certain temptation to stay stubbornly glued to an opinion – after all, you've taken the time to write it down, tweet it and defend it against angry comments. But while you rarely see someone going from right to left wing, or angry detractor to staunch supporter, opinions do evolve gradually. Sometimes a thoughtful comment or response will give me pause for thought, or I'll read someone else's blog and gather a bit more info to go on, or sometimes I'll have a rant to a friend about something, bouncing ideas off them in preparation for writing something. This happens quite a lot with Lucy, who's a brilliant and understanding sounding board for most of my ideas about commitment. If I get into a rant about the pressure to get married and why I hate the very idea of it, she'll gently remind me that there's an ocean of difference between saying 'I don't like it' and throwing everyone who *does* like it under the bus. Which is a good point. When you're so focused on having opinions about everything, it's easy to end up thinking that everything in the world must be 'good' or 'bad'. I did this way more in my early days of blogging: this particular type of sex was The Best, and this other type The Worst. Spanking, throatfucking, threesomes, piss-play: all in the 'good' column. Morning sex, 'lovemaking', anything involving a safe word or someone counting spanks: worst.

Perhaps our sex myths persist because we want to do this simple categorisation for everything. Wherever you look, you can see that humans love a binary: black/white, good/bad, straight/gay, monogamous/polyamorous. And we're so desperate for advice that we'll cling to any shred of help that sounds like a magic formula, that'll help us sort things into this binary right/wrong. My crappy knickers-in-the-air 'seduction style' is just as unhelpful as a candles-and-massage template would be, or a list of 'top chat-up lines', because there is no one single 'correct' answer. Ultimately whether anything works is going to depend far more on what the other person wants than on your particular brand of special sauce, but we don't want to hear that any more than we want our doctor to say 'diet and exercise' instead of 'magic pill'. No matter how much our experience tells us that these things are often down to luck and lust we still demand a solid answer to the question 'how do I get laid?' or 'how do I make them love me?' And just as our desire for magic pills stokes the quack diet industry, so our insatiable curiosity about love and sex means we'll take advice from *anyone* – even people like me, who haven't a clue what they're talking about.

How To Get Over Fear Of Commitment: 8 Steps (With Pictures)

(wikihow.com)

- *Watching* Harry Potter -

Him: If they're that magic, how come they don't have the Internet?

Let's move on: in the process of bringing things to that uncomfortably suburban Wednesday, Mark and I naturally had to move in together. As he surveyed a bedroom, piled floor to ceiling with cardboard boxes, he skilfully established the quickest route to a move-in-day argument.

'We can just leave it all there for now and then move things into the right places as and when we use them, right?'

'No, dearest,' I'm sure I said, reasonably. 'You need to remove the things from the boxes and find a home for them in my... *our* house.'

Our house sounded odd to me. Perhaps not quite as odd as Mark's packing strategy, which consisted of him shouting

'Bin!' or 'Keep!' as I pulled things out of his cupboard. Spare pair of trainers? Bin. Shirts which may come in handy if we ever have to go to a wedding? Bin. Saucepans? 'Bin. That one's still got chilli in, saves us washing it up.' I'd made a monumental effort to ditch some of my junk to make space for his possessions, but it was nothing in comparison to Mark's mega clear-out.

'I don't have much stuff that I actually like,' he explained, hurling clothes, old laptops and other useful things into the 'chuck' pile. At one point a lady arrived from Freecycle to collect his old sofa and expressed slightly too much admiration for the rest of his furniture. She left with the sofa, two coffee tables, a memory foam mattress and a fridge.

'Cutlery?'

'Bin!'

'Pink plastic bucket and spade?'

'Keep!'

'Keep? What for?'

'For when we go to the beach!'

'How often do we go to the beach?'

'We *might* go more. Now we're moving in, it might become our "thing". Put it in the box with the Nerf guns and the Hungry, Hungry Hippos.'

We packed it all up into boxes that Mark, with characteristic foresight, had labelled 'things', 'more things', 'stuff' and 'misc'. Then we cleaned the flat just well enough that we'd have reason to kick-off when the landlord inevitably withheld his deposit, wrestled everything into a battered white van and drove over to my place. Umm, *our* place. It took us half an hour to unload, ten minutes to make a coffee, then at least six months to realise what we'd done.

On that first day, we occupied ourselves by having sex with the bedroom door open, then taking our post-shag appetites into the kitchen to marvel at that most adult of miracles: a fridge full of food that all belonged to us. Solemnly I explained to Mark:

'We can eat anything in this fridge. It's all ours.'

'I know,' he sighed with pleasure. 'You know what's even better? We can *throw any of it away*! No more weird sticky ketchup or half-eaten onion or any of the other things housemates have.'

We high-fived. Next moving-in ritual – Mark introduced me to his coffee-making equipment. Explaining yet again why I was sick and wrong for preferring instant, he gave me very specific instructions on how to use his coffee grinder.

'Beans go in here, yeah?'

'Where do we get beans?'

'Just... from a shop.'

'If we're in the shop already, why wouldn't we just get instant coffee?'

'Fuck off and shut up and listen carefully.' He showed me how to scoop beans into the grinder, close the shiny aluminium lid and begin. Part way through the grinding process, you pick up the half-boiled kettle, pour a bit of water onto – oh, have I not mentioned the ridiculous coffee apparatus? – the ridiculous coffee apparatus, which consists of a paper filter in a whirly cup thing, balanced on top of another cup.

'It's just called a funnel, you dick.'

Then you finish grinding the beans, pour them into the

wet paper thing, then perform a complex ritual of pouring at different speeds and intervals, until it's all filtered through the paper to create a cup of strong, bitter, shitty-tasting coffee.

'*Delicious* coffee.'

'Whatever.'

Living together is pretty great, especially during that initial phase of nesting where we get to decide who gets which drawers and I can revel in an almost sexual thrill when I see his video games nestled next to my books on the living room shelves. For a few months, high on the joy of being able to say 'ours', we do everything that other couples do: cook together, choose which posters we're going to put on the walls (framed, obviously, because we're adults now and we have to pretend it's 'art') and embark on ambitious DIY projects which we will never truly finish. We tackle the slightly overgrown garden, cutting and trimming and mowing and consulting and making elaborate plans until eventually – ta da! It's done. Standing in the ugly and desolate wasteland we've created, we realise we're not quite cut out for this and retreat to the living room sofa.

And, of course, we fuck. In the bathroom, in the living room, at any point in the hallway where there's a doorframe for me to brace myself against. We perfect our casual seduction style until we have everyday sex down to two lines and a five-minute quickie:

'Fancy a shag?'

'Yep.'

Then he slides forward a bit on the sofa, unzips his trousers, and I sit on his cock. Sometimes he'll stick some porn on TV, so we can both watch it while we shag. Like discovering a fridge full of food that's all ours, we get stuck into the other joys of couple-living too: loud sex toys, midnight banging and porn nights on the big screen TV in the living room.

There are downsides to moving in, though, and they're generally the ones that come with any kind of commitment. They're those conversations – I'm sure you know the ones – that begin with a relative asking something a little like this:

'Do I hear wedding bells?'

'When are you going to... you know?'

'Do you think he's going to propose?'

This would be less frustrating if it weren't for the fact that, right up until the day Mark moved in, the question had simply been 'when is he going to move in?' Lesson learned: you can't make the questions stop just by doing the thing people are asking about, because there will always be another step afterwards. While Mark and I were just excited about living together (we've halved our bills! More money to spend on chocolate and Netflix!) others were viewing it as the first step towards something more. Weddings were one thing but oddly the thing that seemed to concern my dad most lacked even the romance of a big white dress.

'What do you *mean* you don't have a joint bank account?' You might remember that my dad is quite a traditional guy. So to him, any kind of romantic partnership should involve the immediate and total merging of all your assets, and a subsequent lack of accounting just to prove you're serious. No 'I'll get this meal, baby' or 'could you give me your half of the gas bill?' – everything should go straight into one pot.

'When I was with your mother, all my money was hers as well. What kind of commitment is it when you're still working out who owes who money?'

'Umm... the kind we like?'

I've had this conversation upwards of 20 times and I can tell you exactly how it goes. Dad says 'merge your money', I say 'we don't want to', he laughs, then offers a lecture on why money's not important: it's about sharing. I know this 'dump everything in one pot' plan works well for some couples. They don't keep tabs on who's paid what, they have a genuine conception of the idea of household income, and presumably they get an extra fizz of that payday delight – your balance has just gone up, but twice! So what's not to like? Let me explain.

For a start Mark and I earn vastly different incomes. Company X pays OK, but Mark's job involves making computers do things (unlike him, I am kind enough to avoid boring people with technical terms) and, as such, he gets paid far more than I do. If we were to put it in one pot, two things would happen:

1. I would resent every single purchase he made, even though realistically they were all being made with his money so it's none of my sodding business. He, meanwhile, would be urging me to buy things I don't need, which I would never end up doing because...
2. I would hate the idea of spending money that wasn't mine, so I'd stop buying anything other than the very basic necessities: tampons, toilet roll, and the occasional bag of supermarket-value pasta to give me the energy to haul myself on the next meagre shopping trip. I'd then stare forlornly at whatever ridiculous bullshit – robot dog, textured keyboard, second Playstation – Mark had

just bought, seething with a combination of unnecessary envy and illogical resentment. Yay sharing!

This explanation doesn't go down well with my dad. At a family get-together shortly after Mark and I had moved in, my sister invited us all to toast the good news. My dad, instead of raising his glass, simply grumbled: 'What are we celebrating? They're basically flatmates.'

The next time I visited my mum, I tried to test her thoughts on it. To get her on my side, I was banking on her natural instinct to disagree with anything my dad had said (because people who are divorced always feel like they have to do that), and the fact that she isn't the most traditional person – she and my stepdad are still not married, despite having been together for the best part of 15 years. I've never asked why, I assume it's because they've both been married before and can't see the point in doing it a second time around. Despite the odd joke from older relatives about 'living in sin', no one seriously suspects either of them of being a determined virgin, waiting for a certificate before they hop into bed. It's another of the things I like about their relationship: their certainty that they don't need to be married makes their love feel, paradoxically, more secure. They are as united on this front as they are on the other things that are truly important to them, like being vegetarian or getting an answer right on *University Challenge*. My mum and stepdad will bicker endlessly over the little things like crossword answers ('Red fruit.' 'Strawberry?' 'Seven letters.' 'Strawbry?' 'Oh fuck off.'), but when it comes to the important matters they're both on the same page. Unfortunately, I forget that despite not being wholly traditional in the way she goes about it, my mum's still quite emotionally attached to the idea of commitment, as I discovered when I tried to get her on side with the 'financial independence' thing:

'I just like my independence,' I whinged.

'Oh, but you know,' she replied cheerily, pouring me a glass of wine. 'Sometimes you just have to give up a little bit of that to show someone you're really serious.'

'But... the reason I'm seriously into Mark is that he doesn't *want* me to give up my independence.'

That was a mistake. She immediately melts at the mention of Mark.

'I know, isn't he brilliant? He's just so great for you. And you know how much he wants...'

'Don't say it.'

'Children.'

'We were just talking about money.'

'I know, but it's all part of the same thing, isn't it?'

'We're going to need more wine.'

It's particularly tricky to break this issue down with Mum because my desire – no, *need* – to be financially independent is a value she taught me herself. When she and my dad got divorced, she was hit with the sudden realisation that spending ten years of your life raising children isn't the most helpful thing to put on your CV and, in fact, frequently leads to patronising employers trying to decide on your behalf whether you can juggle the demands of a job and a life outside it. Consequently, after the divorce, she had three kids, a pile of bills and no sodding way to pay them. Like most single parents, she struggled: bought shitty supermarket baked beans, invented weird new meals made from whatever she could scrape from the back of the cupboard and raised all her kids to prefer the cheapest version of everything (hello instant coffee!). What's more she spent hours sobbing over a tedious sales job, which she'd taken to try and upgrade those beans to ones from the 'not quite so basic' range. She never said it outright, but we took home the message: never be financially dependent. There are some people, of course, for whom it's an impossible dream: whether through illness, disability, childcare or what have you, there are lots of reasons why you might have to rely on someone for rent and bills. But my mum's sudden plunge into life without Dad taught me that if I'm lucky enough to be able to work, I should. Earn money. Have savings. Know I'll be OK alone. Never throw my lot in with someone who could leave tomorrow, stripping me of whatever control I may have thought I had.

Oooh, I sound like a bitch, don't I? If it makes it any better, Mark thinks so too, although he'd probably put it more diplomatically:

'It's only money, you knob end,' he'd explain. 'I'm buying you dinner, not taking away your vote.'

Don't get me wrong; the offer of dinner is always going to be pretty tempting. Company X is becoming a hell of a lot more stressful, and now the blog's more popular I'm getting requests from people to write sex-related things for money. It's essentially always been my dream to be contacted by editors out of the blue, and asked to knock out a few hundred words on the Top Ten Ways To Wank When You're Working From Home, so naturally I can't refuse. But combine that with the need to churn out blog entries every few days, write my first book and respond to the deluge of cock pics and flattering-yet-terrifying requests for advice, I'm starting to find it a bit tricky to cope. Catching me during one of my frequent panics, Mark rests a calming hand on my left buttock and suggests, tentatively, that I could always think about giving up my job? And maybe let him pay the mortgage for a month or so, just until I work out something better?

I won't lie: I let out an actual growl.

Sorry if I sound a bit militant on this topic: I intend to sound *incredibly* militant. Because financial independence is really important to me. Not in the way that homophobia is important to the Westboro Baptist Church: I'd never want to force it on anyone else. But it's not a decision I take lightly: I'm fully aware that if Mark's happy to give me money, then rejecting it makes me sound like a spoiled brat and I'll have to consistently repeat that brattish rejection any time someone nudges me and explains that there's 'No shame in letting your boyfriend support you'. There isn't any shame in an individual wanting this, but there are two dodgy assumptions when you try and push that shit on others:

1. The assumption that in life, all any of us wants is to buy more things and
2. That as a woman I should be pleased when a gentleman wishes to provide me with those things.

I understand the first, and I'm not going to be one of those twats who says that money can't buy happiness: the people who say that are usually rich. While they can understand that their yacht hasn't brought them to a spiritual ecstasy, they usually can't comprehend how miserable it is to have your house repossessed. Money contributes to happiness, but happiness needs other stuff too. For me it's about goals: I set myself a goal, achieve it, and then tiny gold coins of delight pour out of the dopamine fruit machine in my brain and I pop down the pub to celebrate. I don't always achieve the goals: sometimes the happiness machine's in deficit because I spent too much time eating cheese and not enough time working. Still, when I work and earn money, the happiness comes from a combination of the numbers in my bank balance, and the knowledge that I've earned it myself.

It feels weird having to explain this – you never hear men banging on about how important financial freedom is to them. Those who think it's odd that I'd reject Mark's offers would be unlikely to think the same if the roles were reversed. When I was with Adam, I earned more than him and people bit their lips and wondered if he felt OK about that. Now I'm with Mark, they tell me I'm lucky and that it's a nice situation to be in. They'd never ask Mark to explain why it matters to him that he can support himself on his salary. Unless they've actually experienced financial dependency (unemployment, illness and what have you) most men in our culture will never have had to consider it. Because they're raised to believe that they will never be dependent on a partner, they value independence the way we generally value oxygen: it's important when you think about it, but we tend to take it for granted.

No matter how sober I am when I explain this to my mum, though, I'm still shocked when she casually invites me to throw my lot in with Mark. It's not really a 'turkeys voting for Christmas' situation, it's more like one of the Christmas turkeys came back as a ghost in January and urged next year's birds to vote for it too. 'It happened to me, mate, but it'll be different for you – honest!'

It's a bit of a let-down, when you're happy, to realise that there'll always be a new thing you're expected to do or say. You may get to the age of 30 and feel like you've smashed assumptions, rejected the 'traditional' route to happiness and committed to having wild and sexy fun with someone (or more than one someone) that you really like. But there'll be plenty of people poking their nose in to ask you what the next step will be. You might be happy, but there's no 'ever after' on the horizon until you've ticked off the key things on the Life List. Whether it's marriage, a mortgage or a tiny mewling child. Anything that signifies the fulfilment of your expected role: as a wife and mother, or the man who feeds and clothes her. You might want to say, as I tried to, 'we're happy here, let's stop now!', draw a neat line and write 'THE END' in flowery lettering just to hammer the message home. But you can't escape the questions: 'are you going to get married?' 'you'll change your mind about children!' Write your own story all you like, but people will always nag you for an epilogue.

I can't blame my mum, though, and it's not like this chat will end in me storming out shouting 'I will not succumb to your societal norms!' like the stubborn teenager I basically still am. She continues to pour wine as fast as I can drink it, join me in shouting insults at my stepdad while he plays guitar in the corner and I'll never stop asking her for advice, even though we'll disagree, because that's how the world works. If you wanted to know how to build a bridge, you'd ask someone who'd already built one. Likewise with sex and love, your parents have already done it (with at least a partial degree of success) so it seems only natural that they'd have a helpful response. Unfortunately, they fall into the same 'advice' trap that everyone does: they want you to live life the same way as they have. Can I blame my mum for telling me to do what she did? After all, I'm so keen on my own lifestyle that I've written a thousand blog posts justifying my decisions, even when I'm still wavering.

Did I say 'my'? Sorry. I keep doing that. I should say 'our' decisions. Because after a fair few offers, Mark cheerfully relents on the whole 'financial independence' thing, and restrains himself to a couple of eye-rolls if I insist on getting the cheap takeaway because I can't afford to split a pricey one. Realistically, there are far more important things for us to genuinely disagree on, so we get on with the important business of wholeheartedly disagreeing on the other life steps.

Mum's hints about children don't come from thin air. Mark's life plan, so far as he has one, involves fatherhood at some point in the future. Tiny soft onesies and midnight cuddles and proudly sticking crap pictures on the fridge: his ideas around being a dad are similar to what my own dad used to look for, albeit with more Xbox and less camping. On the other hand when *I* imagine having babies, all I see is a sea of vomit. I don't let myself dwell any further, lest I remember what an episiotomy is. When I was with Adam I pictured our offspring – adorable combinations of his best features and mine, with our personal flaws miraculously bred out to leave only the more interesting, less fucked-up elements of our incompetent adult selves. It was a luxury afforded by the fact that he didn't want any, so any potential child could stay firmly in the realm of fantasy. With Mark, the possibility is more concrete so I have no picture at all: the baby is just a ball of squishy flesh. An 'it' – as terrifying as it is tiny. I've gradually moved from an early-20s 'eww' reaction to small children, to a smushy sigh of 'aaah'. It's not really maternal, though, it's the casual acknowledgement of cute that you'd give to a kitten picture on Facebook: nice, but I'm going to scroll past it now and get back to work. To those who say 'you'll change your mind', I'll nod and smile and say 'maybe', all the while panicking because deep down in my soul, there's a howling gap where my maternal urge should be.

This is unfortunate, because getting pregnant would almost certainly stop the questions (for nine months, at least. I understand that once you've had a baby the next question on the checklist is 'when are you having another?'), and it'd certainly eliminate the only major sticking point between Mark and I. I can cope with his occasional sugar-sprees, that end with the living room floor covered in sweet wrappers like someone just blew up a piñata, and he can cope with those times when I passive-aggressively scrub the kitchen, assuring him in an enraged falsetto that 'it's totally fine!' But children? That's tough, because time – as the tabloids are so keen to remind me – is running out. And if Mark genuinely wants to have children then perhaps the right thing would be for me to tell him to fuck off: for real this time, not just as a cipher for 'I love you'. I can never guarantee I'll want them, all I can do is either stick with him for the selfish reason that he's a stunning person and a truly spectacular fuck, or I can break up with him for his own good, thus turning myself into exactly the kind of dickhead I'm ranting about here: one who makes decisions for other people because they're arrogant enough to think they know better.

It's a pickle, for sure. All I know is that I'm not quite ready to make my decision. Sorry, sorry. *Our* decision.

15 Open Relationship Rules For A Better Love Life

(lovepanky.com)

Me: Would you rather have an iPhone 6
or a threesome with two hot women?
Him: Can the hot women take photos in
low-level light conditions?

It's all very well searching for the 'ideal' relationship, but if you've no idea what's really out there, it's hard to pick the best thing for you. When I was young the only relationships I really saw were those of adults around me and the people on *EastEnders*. As a result I could only conceive of three different relationships: happy couple, unhappy couple and Terrifying Love-Triangle That Would Likely End In Death. The idea of a romantic or sexual relationship that involved more than two people would have blown my youthful mind – like if you'd asked me to imagine cookie dough ice cream before I'd heard of Ben and Jerry's. Now, though, open relationships are far more common, and are openly discussed as a genuine option for people who would prefer not to go down the monogamous route. What's more, like Ben and Jerry's, non-monogamy is available in many exciting flavours. There's polyamory (where you have multiple partners with varying degrees of commitment with different people), swinging (where you shag people alongside your partner), casual openness (which can include things like one-night stands). To be honest, as with monogamy, no simple summary can express exactly what might be involved in any open arrangement: that's up for the protagonists to sort out, ideally over a bowl of whichever ice cream takes their fancy.

On the surface it sounds like a dream: one in which I live in a giant mansion with a stable of willing guys. Dominant ones, geeky ones, creative ones with hard drives full of porn they'd like to re-enact, witty ones to flirt with when I'm bored on a rainy afternoon. Perhaps one man brings me breakfast and a hand job, another takes me roughly from behind while I shower off the toast crumbs, then three more surprise me with a trip to the zoo and a gang bang after dinner in the evening. On a more realistic level, the idea of having multiple partners sounds like a good way to silence the voice in my head that's relentlessly chasing variety. That voice gets louder the more comfortable things get with Mark. Fun though it is to have a lazy Sunday in bed, followed by double-act jokes over dinner with familiar friends, it's hard not to note that they'd be improved with an injection of first-date excitement, or a furtive, horny grope that may lead somewhere new. An open relationship sounds like the perfect way to tick all these boxes. And it *would* be the ideal solution, apart from the tiny problem that I'm utterly terrible at them.

When we first got together, Mark and I were fairly open. And by 'fairly' I mean that I shagged lots of people, he shagged one, and neither of us had quite worked out that wasn't the ideal scenario. Decent open relationships, like monogamous ones, are founded on good communication, which apparently doesn't include me texting Mark at the last minute to let him know that I'm busy with someone else, or getting stroppy during a threesome because I think he fancies the other girl more. These are both things that happened in our early days, and he was patient enough to cling on while I worked out that I'm just not suited to that style.

The first problem is one of practicality: there are only so many hours in the day. Which Mark-allocated time slots would I shuffle for a mythical extra boyfriend – a few hours cuddling on the sofa? Testing a new sex toy and letting him recreate my weirdest faces afterwards? The hours spent playing nerdy card games, burning his trolls with my dragon and shouting 'Behold my power, mortal'? I'm already overwhelmed by the sheer online admin involved in having *friends,* before we get started on lovers: texts, emails, remembering birthdays and divorce parties. That's all compounded by a sex-blogging double life, remembering to post and tweet just enough that no one worries I might have died. All the while I have to remember who does and doesn't know about my secret identity. I'm pretty much permanently knackered, so open relationships look a bit like nightclubs to me: I'd love to be able to enjoy one but I think I'd rather have a nap.

Then comes the bigger hurdle: jealousy. Let's be honest, we are *trained* in jealousy throughout our whole lives. Those fairy-tale romances, alongside their marriage myths and happy ever afters, also give us some pretty specific notions about 'ownership'. We're told, from a young age, that monogamous relationships are the only way to go, and that along with those come certain rights over who the other person does or does not get to fuck – an icky kind of possession that goes hand-in-hand with the 'my' of 'my boyfriend'. Mark is 'mine' and I am 'his', and while neither of us is really comfortable with that, nor willing to claim ownership on anything other than half the duvet, I'd be foolish not to recognise that these ideas are influential. Making the leap from that story to the understanding that no one else has an absolute right over your sexuality can be quite tricky. Some people utterly nail it, like a very good friend of mine who has one steady lover and a few others that she sees less regularly. Her primary lover will pick her up from the hospital after an operation, or tie her to the living room coffee table and make her come three times before dinner. But he'll also smile as he watches her fuck other people, or give her advice on how to reply to a Tinder message, offering support and encouragement as she explores the things she does when he's not there.

Before Mark, there was a guy who very nearly helped me get to this magical place. He wasn't simply tolerant of my libidinous whims, he actively encouraged them. The idea of welcoming me into his house after I'd been fucked raw by a stranger turned him on. It's called cuckolding: the most ridiculous word for one of the hottest fantasies. That gut-punch of arousal combined with the thud of jealousy creates a pretty horny mixture and culminates in the ultimate hit of sheer, masochistic lust. He used to masturbate thinking about me with other men. I'd tell him stories while he gripped his aching cock and as I talked about what I'd do to the guy, I'd tease my wet fingers around his nipples as he let out a tortured moan. In the fantasy, he'd be nearby while I was with the stranger. Not in the room, perhaps: outside, waiting. Hearing muffled grunts and squeals as the other guy fucked me in ways he could only imagine. Leaning close to the door to hear the words we'd mutter to each other: Fuck me. Yeah. That's it. That's *good*.

One day I visited a friend for dinner. Well, a bit more than dinner, but we ate to be polite. After we ate, he gave me what I'd really come for: hard, harsh smacks with his hand, followed by a flurry of stinging whacks with a slipper. The build-up to the intense pain as he lifted my skirt, pulled my knickers halfway down my thighs, and whipped my exposed flesh with a wire coat hanger. Delicious torture, delivered with a straight face and an unwavering, solid erection. When I'd borne as much of the pain as I needed to get me slick and trembling, he unzipped his trousers and pulled his dick out, holding it barely an inch from my mouth.

'Now my turn.'

And I gulped him down eagerly, like this was my special treat for being good. I could feel the burning stripes left by the wire on my bum even as his cooling spunk hit the back of my throat. I savoured all the details to tell my cuckold boy ten minutes later: he was waiting outside in the car.

It's too much to ask of Mark, this. Far too much. The cuckold kink is rare, and while it definitely involves the kind of dark, taboo sex I love, it's very different to being 'poly' or 'open'. Open relationships are about rejecting our notions of sexual ownership; they exist *in spite of* our norms: cuckolding is there *because* of them. If there was no taboo about non-monogamy, my kinky boy wouldn't have been turned on by me getting beaten by someone else. He'd have picked me up out of the goodness of his heart, rather than the urgent desire to have me sit next to him with my skirt round my waist. Telling him stories and daring him not to look as I frigged myself in the passenger seat all the way back home.

Mark's take on open relationships is, inevitably, sensible and calm:

'You want to fuck other guys? Well *I'd* quite like to shag April off of *Parks and Rec* - we don't always get what we want.'

Mark agrees that polyamory is far too much hassle and he considers cuckolding to be about as sexy as swallowing forks. He's far more realistic about how we'd handle openness, given my aforementioned brushes with jealousy and the way I ruined our first threesome by crying because I wanted his cock to myself. When pushed he'll admit that a threesome with a guy may well have done the same thing to him. In an ideal world, we'd magic this jealousy away and give ourselves infinite time to carry out extra love affairs. We could live happily ever after – perhaps playing our nerdy card games as a foursome with April from *Parks and Rec* and the guy who beat me with wire. But no matter how tempting, Mark and I just aren't suited to open relationships. I find it far easier to empathise with friends who've had a brush with jealousy than to get my head around those who don't feel it. Neither of us is right, we're just different.

A friend of mine who was in an open relationship tried to explain it to me in terms of emotions rather than physical acts. I couldn't work out how cheating in an open relationship was possible.

'She cheated on you?'

'It wasn't cheating. I don't own her vagina – she can shag whoever she likes.'

'So what did she do?'

'She lied to me. I found out later, and I don't get why she didn't just tell me.'

It wasn't the act that mattered; it was the breach of trust.

I can see why he was pissed off, but at the same time I'm amazed that 'pissed off' was the extent of it. I'd have been a howling, sobbing, whining wreck, and it would have taken months of soul-searching before I could talk about it so casually.

What's more, unlike him, I *did* understand why she wasn't up front about it. The dark, pervy part of me gets it wholeheartedly: there's something illicitly fun about cheating. A fuck that you have with permission is different to one that you have without. The heart-pounding, clit-thumping *naughtiness* of it ticks the same boxes that cuckolding ticked for my kinky boy. It's transgressive. Sexy not *despite* the fact that it's wrong: because of it. In the case of my mate, the lie wasn't there to help her have sex, it was there to make the sex worth having.

Polyamory and swinging can be awesome, just as leaving my other half in the car while I got beaten by a fuck buddy may be one of the best things I've ever done. But it's also a bit like marriage – no matter how many evangelists tell you it's the best way, it's never going to be for everyone. After all,

Malaga is only the best place for a holiday if you like sun, sea and sangria. Some people are more suited to partying in Thailand (Dave), or cycling in the Netherlands (me), or doing road trips across the States in ancient Cadillacs with a back seat big enough to shag on (OK, maybe this one really *is* everyone, depending on who's driving the Cadillac). The desire to evangelise about one style of living isn't confined to my parents or opinion columnists: we all do it. I'll occasionally catch myself nudging Claire to find a nerdy boyfriend like mine. One with big hands and a thick cock, computer skills and a penchant for eating Shreddies at one in the morning. Like a hypocritical twat I'll tell her to change her dating profile and avoid the men who she thinks are smooth and charming. 'Nerds,' I tell her before I realise what I'm doing, 'are just better.' Then I catch myself, realise that there's only one Mark in the world, only one Claire, and chances are Claire would rather spend the rest of her life alone than spend five minutes playing geeky card games, even if she did get to play with my dragon deck.

Occasionally I get comments on the blog recommending polyamory, or – in search of an elusive formula that may work for Mark and I – I'll read through other people's blogs to see how it works for them. Mostly it's like looking into a shop window filled with things I can't afford. Lovely, but fruitless. Sometimes it's frustrating, with people who are polyamorous telling me it's 'natural' or 'the only way'. Polyamorous people evangelise just as monogamous married people do, and while it's more understandable, it's no less annoying. Quite laudably, they're pushing back against the expectation that we should all be monogamous, and in exchange they get a lot of shit from people who don't want to change the status quo. Unfortunately, as they push back against these things, some of them push so hard they topple a bunch of us over. Claiming that any human behaviour is 'unnatural' because we don't see it in the animal kingdom smacks of evolutionary bullshit. Sure, not all animals are monogamous. But not all animals write poetry or watch *Question Time* either. Animals fuck, fight, eat, and occasionally do clever things like web spinning, but humans are so much more than that. We sit in circles at book clubs discussing what we thought of the key themes in *Gone Girl*. We dress in historical costume and re-enact battles of the past (I say 'we' loosely here, but whatever floats your boat). We write sarcastic poetry to entice our partners into doing their share of the housework (Actual note on my kitchen side right now: 'Roses are red/The kitchen is dirty/You know how to clean it/For fuck's sake, you're thirty'). The very fact that we can argue about which kind of relationship works best for us is evidence that there's more than one way to do it. Apart from anything else, the 'natural' argument could be easily applied the other way round. I'm sure my parents could find an example to support their 'get a joint bank account' advice – pointing to species of bonobo that set up home in the jungle, cementing their commitment by pooling their supplies of fruit.

When I've written about this on the blog I've had commenters describe monogamy as 'controlling', which I think is a more interesting thing to consider. One of them explained that it's just as strange to control your other half's sex life as it would be to control their friendships. You wouldn't tell them who they can and can't go to the cinema with, would you? So why would you tell them who they can and cannot fuck? I think it's very different, though, and the answer lies in whether you're 'demanding'. Sure, it's incredibly controlling to insist that your partner doesn't go out with friends, or have any joy in their life other than you – if your partner is like this, there are people you can talk to if you want to get out. But crucially, monogamy when it's healthy is rarely a demand: neither Mark nor I has said 'You can't do this'. Through a process of elimination, experimentation, discussion and mutual masturbation, we've established that our monogamy works best when we can share fantasies without the terrifying stress of ever having to act on them.

'Fucking hell. I mean, fucking *hell*.' We're sitting at a tiny, secluded table in the back of a burlesque club, and Mark is observing the waitresses. Tight corsets, stockings, suspenders, ruffled panties that show off the curve of their bottoms.

'Do you fancy all of the waitresses, or just that one in particular?'

'Both. That one in particular.' He gestures at a slim, punky brunette with a phenomenally gorgeous arse. 'And I also fancy *all* of them. What if *all* of them fancied me back? Wouldn't that be brilliant!' Mark's taste is broad. He rarely gets a crush on individual people, as I tend to do when a particularly hot comedian makes a dirty joke in my direction: Mark fancies almost all of the women. If they are wearing ruffled knickers in a burlesque club, or yoga pants in the park, or a summery dress that drapes neatly over their bottom as they go up the escalator on the tube: all the better. He's not an ogler: one of those creepy guys who stares over the top of his sunglasses, or mutters 'nice tits, darling' as he walks past you – just loud enough that you hear but just low enough that no one else does, so you have to face the walk home burning red with embarrassment and questioning your own sanity. Mark is the kind of person who notices a lovely bottom, then quickly looks away for fear he'll be mistaken for That Guy.

So, as he turns his chair slightly away, worried that people will think he's a sleaze, I try to make him slightly less uncomfortable.

'Which one would you pick, if you weren't already with me?'

'Honestly?'

'Honestly.'

'Whichever one fancied me. Which of the guys in this room would you pick if you weren't with me?'

I have a look around the room – there are a whole bunch of different guys in here and very few of them are dressed like the waitresses, more's the pity. There are older guys in suits looking a bit classy and dashing, with dates they've obviously taken for pre-dinner cocktails. Media types, with skinny trousers and oddly Victorian facial hair. Guys who look adorably nervous, sneaking the same kind of awkward appreciative looks at the waitresses as Mark does. Fat guys, skinny guys, older, younger, gay, straight, attached, single.

'Honestly?'

'Honestly.'

'Whichever one fancied me.'

I don't think either Mark or I would pick monogamy, in an ideal world. We'd both have some version of the mansion-full-of-lovers that I visit sometimes in my dreams. But just as no one gets a freezer full of Ben and Jerry's just by asking for it, so sometimes your dreams just can't work in reality. An open relationship would give us the opportunity to try to get with some of those hot burlesque attendees (although I doubt Mark would want to be 'that guy' who asked the waitress for her number any more than he'd be the catcaller in the street). But if it were possible, and permitted, for either of us to fuck other people then the joy of these conversations would lose their spark. Far from being a fun way to pass the time while we waited for our drinks to arrive, the whole thing would take on a terrifying reality: the need to go and have an actual conversation with a stranger in order to make something happen. The knowledge that most hot strangers turn out to be bellends when you talk to them anyway. The realisation that, sure, I could go and fuck that dapper be-suited cocktail-drinking gentleman, but if I did I'd miss out on that train journey home, where Mark lay his head on my shoulder, and breathed hot, whisky-smelling breath into my ear.

Perhaps the temptation to tell people how to live their lives comes at exactly the moment you find something that works. Because when it works, it feels instinctive: like the desire to pull your hand away from a burning flame, or run screaming from an angry tiger. When instinct draws us towards a particular kind of relationship, it feels so good and neat and – yes – natural, that it's hard to comprehend why it doesn't feel right to everyone.

So You've Decided To Watch Porn Together

(swimmingly.com)

- *After watching* Secretary -
Me: So which bit of the film did you find hottest?
Him: That bit in the middle where we stopped watching and I fucked you in the mouth.

Luckily for Mark and I, there are other thrills beyond sex with other people. Second only to box sets, one of our favourite hobbies is wanking. When I fancy a wank, I do one of two things: I either fire up some porn, or close my eyes and imagine a group of businessmen passing me around like an exclusive corporate perk. The latter is far more common than the former.

'What's wrong with my porn?' asks Mark, scrolling through screencap after screencap of his 'collection'. And I give 'collection' scare quotes because it feels like more than that. A few films might constitute a 'collection'. A couple of hundred or so, even. What Mark has is closer to a 'stockpile', as if one day there'll be a pornocalypse and he'll have to ration out facials and creampies on a strictly limited rota. There's porn in there that he hasn't watched before. There's porn in there that he'll *never* watch. Other videos may have been viewed for 20 seconds before he's clicked on the next one – a vast array of different people, positions and pop shots, to be dipped into at his leisure. And fair enough – he's one of a generation that hit adolescence just as porn became widely available and a kid in a sweetshop doesn't limit himself just to his favourite flavours. Sometimes – and I find this strangely adorable as well as intensely hot – he will sit in the lounge with every available screen tuned to a different part of the same video. TV, laptop, second laptop, iPad, phone: each one showing a slightly different moment in one glorious, high-definition visual orgy.

Yet when the time comes for us to watch things together, he often draws a blank.

'What about the one we watched last time? With the lady in the red pants?' He flicks through, unsure which one I'm talking about.

'We watched it already, so I probably deleted it. Why would you watch the same one twice?'

'It was... good?' I reply lamely, holding his dick in my hand and fluffing while he picks a couple of options.

'This one's BDSM. You like that.' And he presses play. Two minutes later my mind wanders and I turn away from the screen, using the noises to soundtrack the more interesting things happening in my hands and my imagination. The problem is, I really *want to* love his porn. I adore porn in general, whether it's books, pictures or films starring guys with tattoos and a wicked way of wielding a leather strap. Unfortunately, the vast majority of porn misses out the things I find hottest.

If I'm going to get turned on, I want to see a guy's face – excited and eager. I want to see his dick twitching from soft to hard over the course of a minute or so, ideally accompanied by those sexy gulps he does when he knows he's about to get fucked. I want to see his hands gripping it, his naked body framing it and above all I want to know that he's really fucking horny. What I actually end up seeing in most porn is a gaping cunt, a wailing lady, and a weirdly disembodied cock poking in from the corner of the screen. The guys I see in mainstream porn are, almost literally, tools.

There are much better alternatives, but to find them you have to look beyond the hard drive of your enthusiastically straight boyfriend, who'll get most of his porn from the kind of sites that advertise 'Hot MILFs in your area'. There are female (and gender-queer) porn directors making some amazing stuff that doesn't start with a blow job and end with a facial. There are 'amateur' performers (scare quotes because who the fuck decided that anyone's sex should be called 'amateur'?) who are happy to give you the kind of intimate, filthy detail that they'd usually only share with their partners. I hesitate to call this 'porn for women', by the way. Some time in the early 2000s a few people got together and thought 'Hey, we should make some porn that appeals to women'. They'd recognised that the vast majority of non-gay porn was aimed solely at straight guys and straight women rarely got a look in. Some of these people were out and out heroes: creating hot scenes which show a massive diversity of desire. Others brainstormed what they thought women wanted and just came up with a slightly different porn formula: cheesy scripts, soft-focus shots, and the barest minimum of hardcore fucking. Sex, but stripped of the actual sex: like you're all ready for a night of hardcore passion and some misguided lover turns up with a book of sonnets. It means that 'porn for women' is often a mixed bag. Straight guys often assume that because I'm a woman I'll go for this soft-focus mishmash. While I'm happy to put in the time to find porn that includes actual sex, as well as (gasp) shots of the guy's face as he comes, Mark could scour his porn stash for a thousand years and never find something I'll really get on with.

Understanding this porn conundrum helps answer the 64-million-dollar question for men: 'if women love shagging so much, why do *I* never get laid?' It's another of those blog FAQs, usually asked by guys who are at the end of their tether, having tried and tested all the quack advice ('Neg' women by telling them they're ugly! When you've lowered their self-esteem they're *guaranteed* to fuck you!) and still ended up without a partner. The question's usually a rhetorical one, asked not because they want the answer, but to assert what they think they know: women don't like sex. Proof, if it's needed, is that porn is aimed at men. If women liked sex, more porn would be for women.

Let's flip that around, though. Maybe it's not that we don't like sex, it's that sex is presented as something we won't like: something men do *to* us rather than *with* us. Likewise porn is often *about* us rather than *for* us.

Plenty of women love porn and read/watch it at a much higher rate than the media would have you believe – but so often mainstream porn is produced and marketed almost exclusively for men, so we have to either imagine, hack, or gloss over bits if we want to really enjoy it. Proof: go to any major porn site and take a look at the adverts. Naked women with their tits smooshed together will present them invitingly to you. Hot grandmas in your area will scream 'fuck me!' from the side banners. When you get to the splash screen, the silhouetted person bending over and offering you their arse, unsubtly inviting you to 'enter' will definitely be a woman. Every single one of these things is a subtle nudge to straight women that they're not welcome. Given this, you'd think none of us would bother, but surprisingly *women watch porn anyway*. In the summer of 2015 PornHub released some data about their user base that showed 24% of their users were women. Far from women not enjoying porn, I'd argue that the fact that fully a quarter of PornHub's users are women is proof that we're very keen on porn indeed. Would a straight guy wade through an obstacle course of cock in order to get a five-minute glimpse of the kind of porn he fancies? A guy with splayed buttocks inviting him to enter? Ads for hot DILFs who really want to fuck? We do this every single time we watch. High five, sisters.

Or perhaps not 'high five', of course, because if you're a woman who watches porn then there's always the lingering question: is this exploitative? Is this bad? Is this unfeminist? It's hard to tackle this in the right way – write it off too easily and I'm downplaying an important issue. Give it too much weight and I'm pandering to people who would censor sexual expression because they don't want adults to see tits. The question 'is X feminist?' is applied to so many things – is make-up feminist? Are high heels feminist? Are slippers feminist? How about McDonald's Happy Meal toys

– are they feminist? Feminists clearly need to get their house in order and come up with a list of all the things that are and aren't feminist, otherwise we won't know exactly how to smash the patriarchy. Top of the list: porn. Is porn – or indeed any sexual content such as tits on page 3 of a tabloid paper – feminist? I think the question is a bit of an odd one. I'm delighted that we're mature enough to raise it, but now that we have, let's try and tackle it with a bit more nuance than we've applied to sex stuff in the past.

Asking whether porn is misogynist is a bit like asking whether films are violent or food is salty. Some is, for sure. Some is unnecessarily and gratuitously so (I'm looking at YOU, Tesco's microwave lasagne and Tarantino's *True Romance*) but some is violent or salty in ways which are totally legitimate given the context (Hi miso soup and *Kill Bill*). You might disagree with me on those things and that's fine – it's why we have interesting debates on the nature of anything subjective: art, food, books, or who deserves to win the *Great British Bake Off*. If something contributes towards culture, it'll be open to critique. However, asking whether all of it is X or Y belies quite a significant bias. Usually the people who decry porn as 'anti-feminist' have only ever seen porn of the type I lamented above: the one-dimensional, paint-by-numbers videos that make up most content on mainstream porn sites. I'm with you, to be honest – that stuff is often shit and frequently misogynist. But that's unsurprising: given a fairly misogynist world, in which women are often told that our place is to *inspire* arousal but not *experience* it, it would be a genuinely newsworthy miracle if porn itself were immune.

But is *all* porn anti-feminist? Of course not. There's plenty of porn that celebrates female sexuality, treats performers with respect, and doesn't automatically label anyone a 'cumslut' just because they like bukakke. What's more, there's porn made by and for self-identified cumsluts, who get to decide their own rates, shoot their own scenes on webcam, and throw a big, quim-dripping V-sign up at anyone who'd try and censor their sexual expression. There's also a lot of porn that occupies the grey areas in between. Each and every video, book, picture and audio clip (yes, these exist too – you haven't lived until you've wanked to an MP3 of someone grunting at the point of climax) is worthy of criticism. Each one can be analysed on its feminist merits individually. But putting it all in the same bucket labelled either 'Awesome' or 'Awful'? You might as well ban salt.

Before I get too comfortable here on this fence, let's give Mark a word in edgeways, because a lot of the porn I grumble about is the kind of thing he loves:

'Thing is, mate, I just like what I like.'

'Do you not get bored of all the porn showing you the same thing, though? Just the close-up fannies and hardly any wide shots where you get to see everyone's face?'

He looks at me in disbelief, like I've just asked whether he's sick of wanking altogether.

'No. No I don't. Besides, I think you're exaggerating how bad my porn is. There's loads of good stuff.'

'Do you ever want to watch something different?'

He pauses for a second and tries to remember porn I've showed him. Moments when, like a tedious yet horny suffragette, I've sat him down in front of an ethical, feminist porn flick and stared intimidatingly at him to gauge how hard he gets. He reminds me of a specific scene – two guys giving head to a girl – and nods grudgingly:

'I liked that. A lot of guys could probably learn from it, especially when it comes to technique.'

'See? It's good!'

'But it would have been more fun if it hadn't come with your boring feminist DVD commentary.'

Fair point.

The tricky thing when talking about porn – particularly to straight guys who are fans of it – is that if you do anything other than profess a deep love for all of it, you're going to fall into the 'feminist killjoy' trap. I can't fall into this trap with Mark, because he's a feminist himself. He doesn't wear a badge or anything, he just does what I think a lot of feminist guys do: listen to what women say and then go 'huh, you're right', perhaps applauding every now and then, or stepping in when a bunch of colleagues indulge in sexist banter at lunch. We may well be getting into my personal kinks, but guys who are thoughtfully feminist, willing to listen rather than leap into an argument, are sexy as fuck. Definitely hotter than the guy who thinks that any thoughtful critique is the start of an out-and-out gender war. *That* guy clings desperately to his sexist stereotypes in case a horrifying future comes to pass: a future in which he has to fight for a job against people who are better qualified and he won't get a leg up because he's white, stroppy, and male. It's the latter guy who makes me nervous about criticising porn: just as a feminist can't think a joke is sexist without being labelled humourless, so she can't criticise porn without being accused of censorship.

This doesn't mean that I sit behind Mark while he's wanking, lecturing him on what to watch – although that would be enormous fun and I suspect exactly the kind of challenge he'd enjoy. It just means we can discuss porn in the same way we'd discuss films or TV, showing each other our favourites and slagging off the other one's taste when we feel it's necessary. In private, Mark watches what he likes, I watch what I like, and when we're together we compromise. Most of the time that means I get to watch him wank for a bit before we get down to the main event. If I'm not getting the cock-grabbing and enthusiastic, horny faces from porn, then having a boyfriend who'll happily provide them for me is the equivalent of my own private sex show.

Not all women love porn, but a significant enough proportion of us do that I doubt feminism will eradicate it any time soon. Moreover, I'm not sure it should ever want to, especially as more independent producers and performers are starting to change the landscape to reflect more diverse sexualities and desires. It would be a crying shame if we banned porn just as it was starting to get interesting.

Let's get back to the question: 'If women really *do* like sex, why do I never get laid?'

While this question tells us quite a lot about our questioner (he's probably straight, male, and incredibly horny), it also tells us something about straight *girls* who want to get laid. Namely: if you're a woman who fancies a shag, your first job is to persuade someone that you genuinely want to. Let's dismiss the notion that women never *want* to fuck strangers. While there are plenty who'd like to save themselves for their wedding night, there are also women like me who would rather put a condom than a ring on it. I fantasise frequently about five-minute, no-nonsense fucks: from the hot tattooed guy on the tube letting me slide down onto his cock to the daydream about pulling a guy directly from the bar into the toilets and letting him come in the 'V' of my open-necked shirt. Unfortunately, these confessions are usually met with at least one guy who calls bullshit:

'Oh yeah?' he'll sneer, 'then how come no one's ever dragged *me* into the toilets?'

Apart from the fact that he sounds like an arsehole, the answer is far more complicated. Maybe it's because women are so frequently told not to be 'easy'. Or because we're told we should care more about love. Perhaps because casual sex, like porn, is so often portrayed as a male fantasy – one that begins with a naked woman, and ends with a facial come shot – that it's not always obvious to women what's in it for us. I fantasise about stranger sex all the time, but the reality I'm offered has rarely lived up to it.

Take my shagging-in-pub-toilets fantasy, for instance: let's say the stranger meets my eye, and we connect. He smiles ever so slightly, as if to say 'Yeah, I'm game if you are'. He doesn't sneer 'As *if* you would', or nudge and whisper to his mates 'Look at that slag'. He holds my gaze and it feels like we've got a truly filthy secret. My clit thuds with desire. I nod towards the toilets, and saunter off. I can feel his eyes on me as I walk away. I'm wearing something clichéd – tight, short, and easy to lift up so he can pull my knickers down and fuck me against the cubicle wall. Nevertheless, neither he nor any other guys in the vicinity have grabbed me inappropriately, or smacked my arse as I walk past. He follows me into the toilet, knocks, and I let him in. We fuck. In the knowledge that someone could walk in at any moment, we do it quickly. His hands are all over me, doing exactly what I like, which he knows by instinct – it's fantasy, remember? His dick's hard and eager. Without whining or trying to sneak it in bareback, he neatly rolls on a condom, and I bite his neck as he lifts me up onto his cock. He makes the faces he's always wanted to make when he really lets himself go. He grunts. He moans. He fucks harder and I feel him start to tremble. I spit into my fingers and rub at my clit to make sure I get to come tight and hard around him.

Afterwards, when we pull our clothes back down and wander out to the bar, we're both sated and neither is ashamed. There's no high-fiving, no insistence on a post-shag date, no look of disgust or regret in his eyes. We nod respectfully, like opponents in a tennis match, safe in the knowledge that both of us won. That's the kind of stranger sex I want, but it's heartbreakingly rare and not just because pub toilets are always far too crowded. It's rare because we're taught to accept a *male* fantasy of casual sex: one in which guys 'win' something from us that we're not meant to give up and in which all the pleasure exists in that three-second spurt at his climax. A bit like our conception of what porn involves: pliant women submitting to be ploughed in every hole then jizzed on when the guy gets tired, so casual sex is portrayed as something in which all the pleasure is in the scoring and the squirt. Well, bollocks to that. In *my* casual sex fantasies, I have a good time too: orgasms, happiness, safety and ideally a pint afterwards while I enjoy the delicious sensation of a post-fuck pair of wet knickers. Maybe pervy girls like me *could* have all the sex we want, but if the type of shag on offer ends with shame and disappointment instead of pleasure, it isn't going to be a tempting prospect. Like being offered free rein at an all-you-can-eat buffet, but some fucker's burnt all the food.

Science Proves Once And For All That Women Want Sex As Much As Men Do

(mic.com)

Me (sexy face): Are you coming to bed?
Him (sad face): Might as well. The Xbox controller's flat.

'See that guy?' She looks. In fact, we all look. Subtly, you know – we crane our necks almost a full 180 degrees, as if we've all simultaneously wondered where the toilets are. Immediately we recognise the one. He's tall, ever-so-slightly bearded, in a way that pretends to be casual. He's wearing a short-sleeved shirt and a thick wristwatch on his right arm. He's not my type – too toned. But three of them make a guttural 'mmm' noise of appreciation.

'I would.'

'I would too. Twice. Then once again while we're waiting for the taxi.'

We occasionally compete to outdo each other. That one? I'd clone him for a threesome. This one? I'd fuck him down to a *paste*, mate. And if you overheard it, it might sound somewhat intimidating. Like we've been possessed by the spirit of those guys who shout out catcalls, we've just lost our voices so most of it's confined to whispers.

Here's the deal: if someone thinks women don't perv, then they haven't met many women. Or – and we'll get to this later – the women they've met are ones who aren't comfortable doing it in front of them. It's either a strange quirk of life or a genuinely fascinating situation that most sex bloggers are, in fact, women. If we really were sex-averse creatures, why would so many of us be writing about it? The people who ask me 'where are the dirty girls?' rarely stop to consider how strange it is that they're aiming their query at a sex blogger. It's like standing in front of a white, one-horned horse-like creature and asking where the unicorns are.

Women do perv. We are horny. Not all of us – there'll be asexual women, as there are asexual men, but by and large most of us enjoy some form of sexual life. Many of my female friends – and I admit that I'm a skewed sample because I've met quite a few of them via the sex blog – are just as keen to fuck as they are to cuddle. Some of them write blogs of their own, watch porn, or have to cross their legs when they see two hot guys making out on the tube. We don't put on our sexy face just for a man, then peel it off like a mask when he walks out of the door. We drink, we dance, we flirt, and we fuck. And anyone who asks where we are is simply not looking hard enough.

But to write the question off that easily is cheap. There *are* differences, and I'd be dishonest if I didn't admit that. Men visit sex workers in far larger numbers than women do.

Craigslist ads for 'no strings attached' tend to be written by men. While women on dating sites will be inundated with dick pics and lazy chat ups, men rarely receive messages from skeezy straight women with a picture of their cunt and the subject line 'fancy a go lol?'

Perhaps the problem is that the risks often outweigh the benefits.

It's roughly 8pm on a Saturday night and the doorbell rings. In my head – this doesn't happen in real life. But in my head, the doorbell rings and Mark goes to answer it. Standing on the doorstep are four guys. I can't make out their faces, and I don't really need to: fill in the blanks with whichever faces you most fancy licking right now. They're dressed relatively casually, but each of them looks wolfish and eager. Hungry for a fuck. One or two have semi-hard erections pressing against the crotch of their jeans. Mark lets them in. Again, because this is fantasy, he doesn't roll his eyes or make awkward chit-chat. He doesn't shuffle uncomfortably before ushering them through to the lounge: he greets them with charm and wit and banter, the kind he'll use on me when we're alone.

They all traipse through into the lounge, to where we have inexplicably acquired a mini-fridge and a decent hardwood coffee table that wasn't bought from Ikea. They grab themselves beers, or whisky (I fucking *love* a guy who smells like whisky), and proceed to get just a little bit drunk. I'm there, but they don't really speak to me. They chat among themselves, and with Mark, *about* me but never to me. Like I'm basically the entertainment.

Which I am.

At about half past the second drink, one of the guys starts touching me. Without breaking eye contact with his mates, he reaches out, beckons me with a finger and I come and kneel in front of him, facing outwards. He slides a hand down the front of my top and grips one of my breasts in his hand. My nipples are rock solid, and he squeezes one hard, as if to test how turned on I am. I close my eyes and let out a bit of a sigh, and that prompts the others to join in. Hands, lips, all over me. Biting at my neck and scrabbling at my clothes as they fight to tear them off me. Mark stands back and watches, making occasional comments about what a good girl I am.

They take it in turns to bend me over the coffee table. Fucking me in my mouth, my cunt, and – spit-lubed and enthusiastic – in my arse. Mark watches them taking their turns, holding his thick cock in his right hand, stroking slowly so he doesn't come too soon. The other guys take what they like: quick, hard thrusts. Squeezes. Thudding twitches as they climax, pumping come in an arc over my naked arse. When the final one's ready, when he pushes himself tight inside me, Mark stands in front of my face.

'Do you want this now too?' he asks, running his thumb over the wet head of his dick. I nod, and moan, as the other guy enters me from behind. As Mark slides his dick into my mouth he croons that I'm such a good girl. That I'm so well behaved. That I'm allowed to come now.

And it's never ever *ever* going to happen. Which is a shame, for me. Probably a relief for Mark, for whom the idea of a real life gang bang sounds terrifying. He'd be up for the sex bit, but having to do the hosting beforehand would send him into a tailspin of panic. What if he didn't have the right brand of beer? What if he made a joke that fell flat? What if the other guys thought him a nerd? In the fantasy he's proud and in control: the owner of everything sexual that I have to give, and the delighted arbiter of who gets to use which bits of me. In real life, he no more owns me than he owns the stray cat from two doors down, and it's all he can do to work out whether Twiglets or Wotsits would be better party snacks for an orgy.

The point of this particular fantasy, though, as opposed to one of the others that pops up in my head to stop me from getting any work done, is that it's one which I've been frequently told is easy to achieve if I really want to. 'You can do it!' shout men on the Internet. 'Just send out an invitation and you'll get plenty of blokes who are happy to help out!' They're eagerly typing their RSVP before I've started compiling the guest list. I get it: they would. If all I wanted was a group of men, I could find them somewhere. But it's not quite that simple, is it? Like my pub stranger, these men need to fulfil far more criteria than just a vague willingness to put their cocks in me. Most of the criteria are negative ones: they need to *not* be creepy. They need to *not* be terrifying. They need to *not* get overenthusiastic and ask me if I've ever vomited blood. This fantasy can't come true, and it's isn't for a lack of willing men, but an abundance of them.

I've known women who have expressed a desire to role-play dark scenarios: like my kidnap fantasy, they want strange men to do things to them while they pretend to struggle. As a fantasy, this is smoking hot and exactly the kind of thing that would press my buttons. But when they explain and say 'this is a fantasy – it's not real, but I'd like to pretend', they're met with eager gents – genuine strangers – who think they're being generous in their offers to fulfil it. 'Tell me where you live, leave your front door unlocked and I'll do it. Friday nights are best for me.' Or the guy who once kindly offered to meet me on Hampstead Heath at midnight. Or the lovely 'Bitch, come to [Name of city] so I can facefuck you' gentleman.

Chances are they all meant well. It's more than possible that none of them were going to chop me into tiny pieces then hurl those fleshbits into the jaws of the nearest dog. On the surface it might seem that I'm as guilty of judgement as others – assuming that anyone enthusiastic enough to pop round for a gang bang could easily hurt me afterwards. But there's so much tied up in this it's almost impossible to unpick it all. Anyone who sees me as excitingly kinky for fantasising about a gang bang can't have failed to notice a few other things too: the messages we're bombarded with about how men are scary and intimidating, physically more powerful than women, and incapable of exercising restraint once aroused. The sometimes veiled but often blatant victim-blaming: when someone is raped or assaulted one of the first questions asked will be 'what were you wearing?' or some other variation of 'did you ask for it?' So a man offering to fulfil a fantasy like this, in the same casual way he'd offer to lend me a fiver, belies a lack of empathy for the potential risks, and therefore makes him seem risky too. Offering to fulfil a fantasy isn't something that only dangerous people do, but if you want someone to accept your offer you need to understand exactly why *you* might be the danger. I might be dangerous as well, of course, it's just that men are rarely given that brief. Just as they're rarely confronted with stories of sexual assault by women, and an aftermath in which a male victim has to justify his decision to walk home at night drunk and wearing tight jeans. So anyone who wants to fulfil a fantasy like this needs to recognise why their offer, while well-intentioned, can never be casual. You need to build trust and show that you understand the risks. Show you know that anyone who shares this desire also shares a significant dilemma: I want this, but it might kill me.

'I want to take you for dinner,' his email says. And I can't help but read a subtext in this request that's not quite a question. 'Then I have an event I'd like you to attend with me.' I shudder a bit. From a friend this could be a fun proposition. From a stranger it reads like a command, and it's not one I want to fulfil.

'I don't meet people who contact me through the blog,' I explain to him, adding tentatively 'I do hope you understand why.'

'Haha lol,' he replies, wittily. 'I bet you get a lot of weird emails! I promise I'm not a rapist though.'

Which misses the point so swiftly and elegantly I almost want to watch the replay. I'm sure *you're* convinced that you're not a rapist. But the fact that you'll instantly extend your promise means you must understand why *I'm* nervous. It means you know that I live in fear of it. You comprehend why I withhold my face, my name and my address. You know that being a woman who openly talks about sex puts me in danger. But you'll never make the connection that you might *be* that danger. No man wants to think of himself like this, yet few men are able to make the leap from understanding a woman's nervousness in that situation to putting themselves in the picture. You could be the nicest bloke alive: my ideal fuck. You could be warm and sensitive and caring and filthy-hot and horny and willing to do all the things that I want. You may well stop when I ask you to, but equally you might not. And you can 'lol' at the thought of other creepy guys, but while you don't take them seriously I can never really trust you.

I ignore his second email, and he pings me again.

'Don't make me send you flowers.'

He doesn't understand why that frightens me.

So when guys ask 'Where are all the pervy women?' the simple answer (we're in the supermarket, pub, park, street) is never going to tell the full story, because it assumes that we're all on equal footing, and that our horniness is limited only by desire and imagination with no risk thrown in. The fact is that while a guy can offer no-strings sex on Craigslist, or accept a random offer to come back with a woman after a night out, any individual woman has to deal with the fact that giving in to her desires might mean anything from social stigma to rape and even death. That's not to say men are never in danger during anonymous hook-ups – they often are – but they're rarely encouraged to take these dangers seriously, and as a result most guys don't. I, on the other hand, have had it drummed into me from birth that the question: 'Fancy a drink?' comes with a whole heap of other questions: 'Do you trust me?', 'Are you certain I'm not going to kill you?' Questions which make a well-intentioned offer sound simultaneously like a promise and a threat.

'Can you piss on me again?' To be fair, I probably could have picked a better time to ask Mark this than when we were sitting on the sofa and about to crack into a new episode of *Orange is the New Black*. He makes a face.

'I guess. If you really want. But we did it that time ages ago and I'm not sure it's my thing.'

'Haha, no worries,' I lie. 'It was just an idea. We don't have to.' And we go back to watching TV. Sex is more fun on TV, anyway. On TV you rarely see the brush-off when someone's knocked back casually for a kink. On TV you don't have to do that awkward thing where you get a bit tipsy then ask someone to wee on you in the bath. Mark did manage it once, though, like a champ. Standing over me and straining to get the stream of urine started – me hot and bothered and smiling like an enthusiastic mother getting her kid to reach the finish line on sports day. It was horny and it worked, but there was something missing. When I'd done it before with other guys, the hotness came less from the piss itself (body temperature, in a metaphorical as well as a literal way) than from the desire they had to defile me while they did it. The 'take this, Bitch', attitude that – from someone I love – makes me squirm with need. With Mark it was more like he was humouring me: putting a valiant face on something in order to make me happy. Which is lovely, for sure: it's love. It's just not quite as horny.

'Who's my weird pervert?' he asks and pats my head. I snuggle up, then spend the next 20 minutes of the programme trying to stealthily work my hand up one leg of his shorts. 'How about a compromise?' he says. 'When I've finished this can of Coke you can watch me have a piss.'

His offer is kind, but humiliat...

'Yes please.'

'Good girl.'

So, that's where we are, by the way – the pervy girls. We're sitting on sofas with blokes we know we can trust, sometimes trying to persuade them to wee on us in the bath. Occasionally we're making dinner with them in the kitchen, complaining about the inefficient way they chop peppers. We're lying prostrate over their knees while they spank us through M&S flannel pyjama bottoms and hoping they'll pull them down to stick in a cheeky finger or two. While many of us are openly kinky, there are plenty more pervy women who'll keep their desires hidden because of the exact same myths that dictate our other relationships. Some girls are afraid they'll be branded sluts. Others might feel strange or abnormal for admitting to desires that are outside the mainstream. Still more will fall into the 'terrified' category above. And the rest of us? Well, we'll be dropping hints, whispering dirty secrets, and winking at you in suggestive ways, but it's tricky for guys to notice if they're too busy lamenting their own unfulfilled desires.

Mark enjoys some things that I don't, but not once has he moaned that I won't fulfil his sexual needs, or that my dirty talk has written cheques my cunt cannot cash. He accepts that you can be discerningly horny, and that an enthusiastic 'yes' to anal one night doesn't mean you get to throw a tantrum if the next time it's a 'no'. Likewise, when I tell him my own fantasies he never reacts with disbelief or shock. He doesn't say 'but girls don't like that!' or 'really?!' in a voice that makes me feel small. He calls me a weird pervert with a grin on his face and a hand down my knickers, accepting that my perving is as much a part of me as my greater skill at chopping peppers.

Where *are* all the pervy women? It's possible that some are reading articles entitled 'twelve ways to get out of sex without using the "headache" line', thinking there's something wrong with them because they aren't searching for an excuse not to fuck. Perhaps they're sitting in the pub, overhearing a guy telling his mate that someone was 'a grubby slag' because she sucked his dick when he asked her to. They might be watching some porn on Xhamster, seeing all the ads for 'hot wives who want to fuck NOW' and wondering if they're freakish for enjoying something that's only for straight guys.

Ironically, every time someone launches into that bitter lament that women just can't be pervy, they're perpetuating the ideas that cause pervy women to stay silent in the first place. We're not unicorns, we're ten a penny, but we're unlikely to come and say 'hi' if we know we'll then have to engage in a heated debate, explaining why we *really* want what we say we want, and we're not just pretending so we can sucker you into something else.

I might be desperate for a hot guy to fuck me in the arse, but I won't go and chat up the one who's spent 20 minutes bitching that women never want it. Especially if that guy (as is often the case) is the same dude who crows about each sexual encounter as if he's managed to steal a precious jewel from the lady in question: 'She totally gave it to me, mate. Gagging for it.' Or – worse – discussion that's evocative of rape and pillage: he 'smashed it' or 'destroyed her'. If you talk about sex like I won't enjoy it, why would I ever expect to enjoy it *with you*?

One of the easiest ways to find a woman who is into fucking in the same ways as you are is to challenge the idea that these women don't exist. You can hang out on chat forums with other straight men, bemoaning the lack of women who want to gobble your cock like a Thanksgiving turkey, or you can get on Twitter and Facebook, join in the talk in the pub and stick up for your fellow perverts – male or female. Challenge the narrative that straight women give straight men sex as a favour. Avoid calling people sluts, or frigid, or tight or anything that implies there's a 'right' and a 'wrong' way to exercise your sexual choice. Don't be the guy who asks whether girls can *really* enjoy spanking, be the one who listens to the thousands of women who tell you they do. Be one of the guys who doesn't slut-shame a girl for first-date sex, who reacts with delight at a girl's kinky suggestions, rather than sceptical surprise that she could ever have had the idea. Be the guy who, like Mark, smiles at the suggestions, working out a way to mesh them with his own fantasies ('want to come and watch me pee?') to create a unique scene of hotness that works for both of you.

Where are all the pervy women? I don't know about the others, but you'll usually find me hanging out with *these* guys.

12 Things That Definitely Do Not Count As Cheating So Please Stop Sweating This Stuff

(bustle.com)

Him: I love you despite you being an arsehole,
but I'd still love you if... you know... you weren't.

'Would you still love me if *I* was a zombie?' We're onto question five in one of our many hypothetical discussions. They usually start with a ridiculous premise:

The world has almost ended, and there are five people left on the planet. You're one: pick the other four.

Then they'll meander through a few lazily horny sub-plots designed to give us a sex break halfway through.

Yeah but really – if you could clone me would you clone me and choose me for all four?

Mark always plays along, because he's good like that. He'll add in a few caveats of his own:

If all four were you, then could I be the king? And could

I have a 'midday blow jobs' rule, or make you all wear hot pants and pull me around on a chariot?

And we'll eventually settle on a healthy compromise.

Midday blow jobs: fine. But we take it in turns to pull the chariot.

Ultimately, though, all the questions go to one of two destinations. The first (and most common) is filthy, and it will end with Mark gently massaging one of my tits while he talks about the fluid dynamics of breast-jiggling and how maybe two of his chariot-pulling clones could run backwards topless. Only two, mind, because the bum-jiggling is also vital. I like this path: it means I get laid. And on a less selfish note, I find out yet more of what happens inside Mark's head. The next time I want to get his dick hard, I'll have an easier go-to fantasy to draw on. When I ask if he likes tits or arse (arse, but it's a close call and ideally he'd like a few minutes to ponder it while staring dreamily into the middle-distance), I'm one step closer to the ultimate Mark cheat-sheet: *what exactly does he like*? It might be annoying when I insist on an answer to something as nuanced as 'is it better to jizz with great volume, or with force?' or when, on the edge of sleep, he rolls over to be confronted by my wide-eyed request that he tell me the last thing he wanked to, but each nugget of information is important. If you ask me what I like sexually, I could write two thousand words that passably reflect what goes on in my head. Mark, on the other hand, would sit in front of a blank page for half an hour and eventually scrawl 'tits' before throwing it in the bin. The questions help the exposition: like I'm collecting pieces of a complex, horny jigsaw puzzle, and when I've slotted the final piece in I'll have a beautiful (and delightfully obscene) picture of the sexscape of Mark's mind.

Sometimes the questions take us somewhere else, though – a darker place, which we don't joke about so openly. The route follows questions like this:

Would you still love me if I couldn't speak any more? (Answer: yes, probably more you mouthy twat.)

Would you break up with me if I accidentally broke your iPhone? (Answer: no.) *If I broke it deliberately?* ('Hey Siri. Text Sarah 'you're dumped.')

What if I cheated on you? (Long pause. Silence. An acknowledgement that this question has no simple answer. The answer is 'It depends' and 'Are you sorry?' and 'Are you planning to?' and a whole host of other things that you can't really get into when you're trying to be playful. When the playfulness masks a very real and direct fear. Eventually a 'Yes'. But not a *real* yes – a deterrent. Like hitting a dog with a rolled-up newspaper – knowing it won't stop the fucker from chewing your slippers again but hoping against all evidence that it might.

I don't want to get too cynical, but all relationships die. Don't let the loved-up passages in this book fool you into thinking that Mark and I will sail easily through to a happy ending: we're only halfway through. You wouldn't celebrate your exam results before you've sat the tests, would you? It's been easy so far because we've only had the fun bits – when challenges come along I'm sure we'll deal with them just as badly as anyone else does. We're only people, after all. And people are useless and weak and they fail.

Remember my stepdad? Singing drunkenly at the piano with my mum, bashing out clunky chord sequences and giggling with her like the pair of them had some kind of magic secret? The guy whose playful dicking-about convinced me that love was something far more akin to a pissed-up pillow fight than a sincere declaration of devotion.

He cheated on my mum. Not in a dumbshit, drunken, impulsive way, either. A full-blown affair: true love, he called it. He'd found someone else who was so perfect for him that he simply had to leave – throwing a pitiful bag of possessions together and disappearing into the night.

Like most bad news, I found this out via a phone call at 2am. My mum was sobbing the way I'd done when my first ever boyfriend had cheated on me. Retching, hiccuping, incomprehensible splutters and those keening moans that you try to hold back, but which burst out of your chest anyway. Bolt upright in bed, I tried to make sense of it. A few words, then a few sobs, then more words. My fear in that moment was that someone had died. Fuck it: that *he'd* died. I went cold with shock at the thought of my funny, loveable stepdad: gone.

He *was* gone, of course, just not like that.

'He doesn't love me any more.'

'What?' I couldn't decipher any meaning from the phrase.

'He doesn't. He doesn't...'

'*Who* doesn't?' And still I didn't get it. Fuck's sake. I'm such a clumsy twat. As if the answer could be anyone *other* than him. As if anyone else's love would be so certain, so immutable, that when it was wrenched away she'd stumble into this bleak pit of sobs.

'He doesn't love me any more.'

That was it. Over and over. Not 'He's gone', but 'He doesn't love me'. The bare fact that he'd gone was sad, but it paled into nothing compared to the more monstrous implication – that he hadn't wanted to be there in the first place. What Mum had enjoyed he'd been enduring: the passion, the jokes, the shared experience, Friday night after Friday night driving neighbours mad with 'I Was Born To Love You' at the piano.

'He doesn't love me.'

On the phone, stammering into the line, the lack of love was all she could see. It was the only thing that mattered – a horrible truth that she was trying to mantra into meaninglessness. Perhaps if she said it enough it'd become just a simple fact, stripped of emotional weight. 'He doesn't love me any more.' A full stop at the end of a sentence rather than heartbreak at the end of the world.

We'll come back to them later, I promise. It's not the end of the world by any stretch, but it's definitely the end of the idea that this kind of love – the passionate, drunken, calling-each-other-twats kind of love – means that any relationship is safe from being smashed into tiny pieces. My 18-year-old notion that romance, if done right, could potentially work forever was just as wrong as all the other things I thought at 18. If I told you that the stepdad incident had happened long before I met Mark, pop-psychologists might shift excitedly in their seats. Maybe this is why I'm so pathetically averse to commitment? Perhaps my unreasonable refusal to settle down and get married has less to do with politics and more to do with fear? It probably does, a bit, but when I think of my stepdad fucking off, it's not Mark I'm scared about. I don't think Mark will leave me, despite his assertive replies to my childish questions. I'm scared that some twitch of lust will mean I'm the one who leaves. I'm utterly terrified by the immutable fact that no matter how much heartbreak cheating causes, for some reason people still do it.

I.

I still do it.

Sex makes no promises. It's not like you fuck someone once and you're bonded for life – there's no contract implicit in the act of orgasm. It's an itch you scratch when you're horny, or a quick fling that seemed fun while someone's dick was inside you, but far too much hassle when it wasn't. Love, on the other hand, makes a promise it can never fully deliver: I'll be here forever. Rock solid and certain and warm and nurturing. It's the sneaky double-glazing salesman of relationships, smarming his way into your house with bold claims of indestructability. Love says 'You're safe with me, because I conquer all. I'm eternal and everlasting'. What horseshit. Sex has at least one benefit over love: while it won't necessarily provide more happiness or last for longer, it doesn't trick you into thinking that it will. When sex shatters and you have to re-glaze your house, you shrug because you knew it'd happen. By the time love is broken, you've been relying on it for so long that it's too late to inspect the warranty.

I've cheated on Mark.

And I saved that for this chapter so you'd have faith in us at the start. So you'd think 'Oh, maybe this'll work out and she's not really the undiscerning horny shitbag she appears to be'. Well, sorry about that, but I am. I am also a predictable shitbag. The kind of person who'll get drunk and beg a hot guy to grope me in a crowded bar. The kind of person who'll call Mark shortly after and tell him I'll be late home.

What counts as cheating? If you've read this far you'll probably be roughly with me: anything that you've reasonably agreed not to do. 'Agreed not to do' because some people *do* agree to fuck others. 'Reasonable' because, well, you wouldn't let hundreds of years of cultural shame about sex dictate what's OK between you and your partner. It's not cheating if you have a wank, because we all do it. And if your partner tells you not to then their request is about as meaningful as if they ask you not to eat while they're out of town on business. A fuck? Cheating, of course, in a relationship like ours where we've decided that the pain would be too much for the other to bear. Beyond these simple extremes there are the grey areas. Is it cheating if I, tipsy on cider and lacking in judgement, get a bit too close to a colleague at the Christmas party? If I light his cigarettes and talk about blow jobs, and flick my hair in a parody of the flirty cocktease? Probably not. That'll just be the beer talking. When I confess it to Mark it will elicit no more than an eye roll and a 'bad girl' and a fuck just hard enough that I could tell he was slightly jealous. More, though: what if that chat led to a kiss – just a little one? One where I stayed just a second too long, reaching out to slide my hand from his waist down to his crotch? Where I could feel his cock pressing gently back against me. Maybe that was cheating. Maybe it wasn't quite cheating, and what tipped it over the edge was when I whispered in his ear that I wished we had a private place to go. Perhaps it would only have been cheating if opportunity had afforded us that place.

Maybe cheating is only defined by forgiveness. Did Mark forgive me? Yes. Therefore there was something to forgive. Not the furtive fuck in an alley, which would have happened if I'd had the chance, but the unspoken knowledge that I was just a lucky interruption away from finding it.

It's not the only time. There have been other forgiven moments. Kisses, mostly. Times when – drunk, always drunk – I'd nod and smile when a guy leaned closer, or I leaned too quickly into him. A quick hand touching lightly under the table. A palm placed firmly on the back of my neck. A hug that went on for too long, and the tell-tale sound of me inhaling the scent of a guy who smelled so different. Good different. *Sexy* different. Not-Mark different. Occasions when Mark wasn't there and his not-there-ness felt like as good a reason as any. If we judge by the wish for something more, I'm a cheat a thousand times over.

Is it only cheating if you enjoy it then? In which case, the brief kiss I shared with a colleague – a scandalously embarrassing kiss, at midnight in a bright train station, in front of a horrified friend – that one wouldn't count. Would it?

The refrain of the regular cheater – does this count? Is this bad? Is this less *naughty* than the last one? Darling, which painful heartbreak hurts you the least? Which of the injuries I've caused you is most easily repaired?

I'm scum.

And yet – at this point, right now, just halfway through – I can honestly say I've never done the worst. Touches? Sure. Kisses? Of course. But shout it from the rooftops in an orgy of misplaced self-congratulation – *I've never slept with anyone*. That pounding, sticky feeling in my chest that tells me I should get away before I do something irreparable: that feeling has so far prevented me from the worst. With Adam, I did. With others, I have. But with Mark? I've never done the worst.

Does that make me any better? Probably not. We come back to what counts. It depends on whether my indiscretions (a delightfully mealy-mouthed word, which covers all manner of selfish, cunt-driven sins) have not crossed boundaries because of opportunity or because of desire. Am I a strong sexual warrior, using the force of her willpower to keep her lusts from tipping over? Or am I, more likely, just lucky that opportunity hasn't offered a convenient enough temptation? With all these words and excuses am I pretending to be sorrier than I am? Because if I'm not sorry – if I don't hate myself enough for any of this – then I'm no better than my stepdad, wringing his hands weakly and saying things that feel even crueller than the act itself: 'It's not that bad'. The ringing horror of those words is rarely obvious to the one who says them. But to the one who hears, the implication of insignificance carries an extra weight: cheating matters less if I never really loved you.

I love Mark. But if love means monogamy then that's almost certainly where I'm failing. Maybe the reason I feel so ambivalent towards romance is that there's a piece of my brain that can never make it fit with what I really want. My cunt and my head don't want different things: they both want to fuck whoever's willing to let them. They also want to be the kind of person who doesn't.

Mark greets each mistake with a kind of weary acceptance, giving me breath-sucking tight hugs, as if he's trying to squeeze the sadness out of me. I'm home late, he's worried. I stumble in, sloppy-drunk and smelling like vodka and shame and chips.

'I did bad things.'

'I thought you might have.'

A pause. A hug. Some tears. A lump in my throat where there should be an apology. He doesn't cry, he just holds me in a way I don't deserve to be held and comforts me. Stroking my head and shushing me as if the whole thing was out of my control. Each time it happens he tells me the same thing:

'I have faith in you.' Which is different to trust, apparently. He has faith that I want to be with him, and simultaneous faith in me being a drunken, horny fuck-up. 'I have faith that you'll always know if you've fucked up, and you'll always tell me.'

'I won't do it again, I promise.'

'OK,' he says, knowing I will.

Then I put on the kettle, and start a now-familiar ritual: coffee. For the next two weeks, I'll make plenty of coffee – hand-ground the way he likes it. After each of my fuck-ups I do this: a penance that's less punitive than it is therapeutic. He knows that I won't be happy until I feel I've been punished, so he allows me to make token gestures of repentance. He doesn't know what I could do instead and neither do I. Maybe if I can't show love by keeping my knickers on I can show it in how low I bow when it's time to apologise afterwards: see how much I love you? I'm grinding coffee while I break your fucking heart.

Why You're Not Having Sex

(*health.com*)

Him: Does this outfit look weird?
Me: No, it's fine.
Him: Oh god I knew it. If **you** *like it then it must be awful.*

Let's put those worries away for now. This is a true story, after all, so let's make like normal people and stash the awful bits somewhere we don't have to look at them. It would be lovely to wallow in emotion while Mark and I have a heart-to-heart, but in reality other things get in the way: work. Life. Sorting through Mark's 'Stuff' and 'Misc' boxes that still haven't been unpacked a full year after he's moved in. All the while I have to pitch, write, make sure that I'm getting a certain number of blog posts live each week or the graphs will go down. I'm not sure why I fear this, but I do. On top of this I have to turn up to Company X every morning or the mortgage won't get paid. The bills won't go out on direct debit. I won't get to moan to Claire about how the boss decided I should scrap a big project then start the whole thing again from scratch.

I'm grateful, at least in part, for the distraction – the idea of having nothing to do is far more terrifying than the idea of fumbling madly through a forest of tasks. At least while I'm in the forest I don't have to look outside at what's really going on. I can just enjoy the occasional spots of happiness, when I don't have to think about anything else.

And of course those occasional spots all involve sex.

'Face the fucking wall.'

I stand, trembling, waiting for him to lock my ankles into the spreader bar, and put me in an off-balance position. It's thin, clinky metal – the sound of the padlocks jingle against the bar as he secures the cuffs around my ankles. And I put my hands on the cool plaster to hold my balance while he locks me in place. I used to think that the point of spreader bars was to keep my legs open: giving easy access and a view that makes him hard. A display that's a cross between arousing and humiliating for me: open and ready for him to touch, to stare at, to fuck. But it's more than that: it's not just about access but *control*.

Spread wide by the bar, every muscle in my legs and back is tense with the effort of staying balanced. Sometimes I'm on the bed, crouched with my face buried in the bedsheets and my back arched in a way I could never hold on my own, arms stretched beneath me to grip the metal. My whole body's twisted in a way that highlights my discomfort and helps me embrace the shivering relief of pleasure as he fucks me with quick, long strokes. Other times, like now, I'm standing up – wobbling on uncertain tiptoes. When the bar is firmly in place, spreading my ankles and my cunt wide for him, he gently but firmly takes my wrists, and places them on my calves so I have something to hold onto.

There's something about being slightly off-balance.

I'd like to say that I don't care if he can fuck me with power and strength: that a gentle shag is as fun as an angry one. But I'd be lying. Especially now, when the rush of the outside world feels like it might just knock me over, when I'm with him I can revel in that feeling rather than fear it. I'm weak and small and vulnerable, but it's OK. I can rely on him to hold me still – hold me *stable* – while he fucks me. Trembling and wobbling and knowing that the only reason I'm upright is that he's got a fistful of my hair.

He stands in front of me and pulls my head back and forth. Quickly at first. Getting the full, satisfying length of his cock in my throat. Down right to the base so I choke, holding me there for exactly as long as I trust him to, then pulling me back. With my wrists and ankles restrained I can't move away. I must stay until my eyes water and he deigns to pull me back – spluttering and drooling and covering him in wet spit. Then more slowly. Holding me in the right position so I can just wet the tip. Licking around the head. Hair straining against his hand and the backs of my knees starting to wobble. And as my legs start to go he pushes me further down, until my face is buried in his crotch, smothered into him so I don't fall over. The back of my throat contracting against him as he calls me a good girl.

I feel more solid on my feet when my face is pressed against him, but it's harder to breathe: a trade-off that he has the power to balance perfectly. He switches me between fast and slow – trembling and choking, secure and nervous. Happy and happier.

When he starts to fuck me from behind, the tremble sets in again. I want to grip my ankles, or lift my hands to hold onto something: the bed, the wall – *anything*. But each stroke of him fucking me makes me tremble harder, feeling like I'm teetering on the brink of collapse. It's relaxing because it's exactly the opposite – tense, tricky. Something that holds my mind in exactly that moment, where tasks and work and emotions matter less than the simple act of staying vaguely upright. Knees twitching in an effort not to crumble.

He likes the twitching, I think. He can feel my muscles tense as he grips me and he can feel me pushing back to take him further inside me – part satisfaction and part safety: the harder I push back the easier it is to stay stable. I think he likes the clinking sound of metal-on-metal too – it means my ankles are still cuffed to the spreader bar, and the rapid tinkling as my legs start to really shake means I'm close enough to coming that he can speed up to bring himself there. Fuck me harder, faster. The swift, angry strokes that give me both release and *permission*. I can come because I know he's about to. The twitching squeeze as I come on his cock brings him to a harder climax.

He grips my hips to keep me upright as he empties himself inside me.

He keeps his hands on me even after he's done – maintaining balance, unlocking me from the spreader bar. I can feel his spunk dripping down the inside of my thighs, and his big hands on my hips. Perfectly balanced, and strong enough to keep me from falling. When I'm unlocked he lets me down slowly – rubbing the soft, wet skin on my thighs with his big hands, and murmuring words into my ear. Congratulating me on staying upright, even though the skill was his. Lying close against me, so I can feel that gorgeous cuddle-temperature-warmth of his body squashing against the entire length of me. When I breathe out, and he breathes in, it feels like he's catching my sigh.

'That was fucking great,' he says. 'We haven't done that in a while,' and I think he means it as a compliment.

We don't fuck like we used to. Sorry about that. I want to be the person who says you can screw like you did when you first met, forever and ever. Bollocks to the people who say sex dies after 60, or that any relationship will inevitably hit a seven-year itch. And I'm sure that's true: sex doesn't have to die. If your relationship is built on a foundation of angry banging, then it's not like the fuck police will turn up at your door seven years down the line and confiscate your libido. Sure, some people shrug and sigh and buy cats, then initiate date nights on a Wednesday as an excuse to throw the cats out of the bedroom and have a half-hearted hump. That's fine. But one of the weird things that comes with our quest for love is the assumption that when you've ticked that box (regardless of the nagging involved with ticking the next one) you can then basically give up on the one before. As if sex is just a mating dance, and once you've shimmied well enough to get someone to come home with you, you can drop the pretence and sit around in sweatpants for a decade. I *do* sit around in sweatpants, of course, I am a normal human. But Mark's got a bit of a thing for tight, faded grey fabric, so they're not the boner-killer that they're often made out to be.

The sex *has* gone south, though, and I don't know why. When he slips into bed with me at night and slides a hand carefully down my stomach and into my knickers, I squirm with discomfort rather than lust. My brain is interested: my brain's *always* interested. My brain would perk up and slick her knickers at the slightest promise of cock. But my body is another matter: it twitches and shifts and refuses to get wet. Mark's fingers, previously borderline magical in their ability to get me hot and panting, now feel clumsy and harsh against me. I used to love his hands. They're big and soft – fat fingers and well-clipped nails and smooth skin and wriggling enthusiasm. Perfect for me to grind against, seeking out his thumb with my clit as he buries his fingers deep in my eager cunt.

Now, though? It's on and off. Some nights it works perfectly, other nights I need more of a push: his soft lips round one of my nipples, teeth giving gentle bites and dick grinding into my hip: then and only then does the wetness flow. On other nights I try and will myself to get wet, feeling like a failure if I have to get the lube. When we fucked before, with hard and vicious strokes, my mind was deliciously blank. Now when we fuck I *think* things:

It's late.

That feels weird.

I'm tired.

Why aren't I wet?

Not like that.

What the fuck's wrong with me?

I used to love that and now I hate it and I just...

I should say.

Fuck.

Just... get on with it.

I've gone from 'get it in me' to 'get on with it' in the space of just a few months, which is worrying. Because if the sex has gone dry and yet we still love each other, does that mean we've hit the brick wall I refused to believe existed? All those people who joke at parties that there's no need to give endless blow jobs when you've already snagged a man, as if the blow jobs I was giving were only ever done for the purpose of tricking him into staying... Are those people right? They can't be. You *can* still fuck after years together. Know how I know? Adam.

Adam and I were together for eight years and in the last of those eight years we had sex exactly as much as we had in the first. Probably more, if I'm honest, because during the first year of our relationship we had to dodge flatmates in shared houses and drink so much student union cider that we were could barely work out which hole to put it in. Was it because we were just a lot younger? I'm older now and naturally my body is starting to do some things that would have horrified 21-year-old me: most notably all the extra places it's started growing hair, and the fact that it has introduced me to the concept of a hangover. Perhaps along with these things comes a steady decline in libido – my cunt's way of saying 'Hey, slow down a bit, it's a school night and there's work to do'.

When I first discovered masturbation my body put me straight into discovery mode: all I ever wanted to do was wank, and in the name of teenage science it was incredibly important for me to work out all the best conceivable ways to do it. Likewise with Adam, my body was keen to explore every single inch of his: from those beautiful dimples just above his hip bones to the bulge and twitch of his prostate.

When he walked into a room I'd feel a powerful desire to sink my teeth into him. Like an angry lioness I'd want to drag him to the floor, haul him up the stairs, then tear his whole body open so I could climb inside. It's considered more polite and less terrifying to offer a blow job though, so that's what I did. Blow jobs and beatings and group sex, weird games with lube and butt plugs, and fucking and fucking and fucking. For eight long years. Never once did I want to just 'get on with it'.

There are a million different ways to say no to sex if you don't want to hurt your partner's feelings. 'I'm so knackered', works well, especially if he can see that you have visible circles around your eyes, and you've spent the last hour sobbing because you're going to miss a deadline. 'I feel itchy' is a weird one, but when linked to the kind of hormonal contraceptive that makes my skin tingle all over, sending jolts of tickly weirdness through my limbs when he touches me: totally adequate excuse. 'Headache', is OK, but then he'll make me feel worse about it by bringing me pills and grapes and cuddles and kindness. Some of the pesky reasons just refuse to come out of my mouth: my cunt's dry and I don't know why because you're doing all the things that should work.

We all have ups and downs, but writing that in black and white makes me feel I've betrayed my Internet persona. Girl on the Net's supposed to be up for shagging all the time, right? That's the impression I get, when I'm tweeting about things other than sex and the only replies that come are a crop of innuendo. If you're a sex blogger, never tweet that it's been a 'hard' day – you'll be drowned in double entendre. When these replies come in I remember recent nights – Mark's fumbling, dry, well-meaning fingers and the ticking panic in my brain as I count down to the moment when I feel like I can't bear it. And I think 'Who *is* the girl they're replying to? I don't recognise her.' I wonder if she ever really existed. I read back over blog posts I wrote before – about the time I persuaded Mark to put a vibrating butt plug inside me so he could feel the buzz along the length of his cock while we fucked. The sound he made when he slipped his dick in, coming almost instantly at the tingle of vibration through the walls of my cunt. And I wonder: was this real? How could this ever have been the most important thing on my mind? Where did I find the *time*? Now my main thoughts are of deadlines. Tasks. Rushing. Achieving new things. Making that bloody graph go ever upwards. And there's a horrible moment where I wonder if that past version of me did all this just for clicks. If I begged Mark for more anal because I knew lots of people Google it. If – eww – I care about him just because no other guy would let me do this. No one else would read my blog posts and think not 'this should be private' but 'This one's cute, I hope they like it'.

That's what he thinks: it's cute. In a way that simultaneously baffles and astounds me, Mark's absorbed my idea of romance. I hand him my phone so he can check on something – a post that contains more violence than normal, the kind of hard-fucking, dangerous fantasy that I'd never think of trying with a guy who wasn't him. And he nods, and understands, and grows a thick erection in his tight jeans as he reads the word 'choke-fuck', before passing my phone back and telling me to publish.

'It's good. I love it. You're adorable.'

And I love *him*. So much. This wouldn't be so terrifying if I didn't – I love him and I simultaneously don't want to fuck him. His body is the same as it was before and it's still beautiful. But the lust it inspires now is more wistful, not 'I want this' but 'why don't I want this?' I feel like taking my own body back to the shop that it came from and asking them for a refund. 'It doesn't work, mate, sorry. What do you mean it's out of fucking warranty? I'm not dead yet!'

After weeks and months of this, he gives up. No more gentle touches or surprising new tricks. No more slipping his hand down the back of my knickers late at night, and holding himself tense as he works out whether I'll embrace him or bat him away: eventually Mark gives up too.

'It's fine,' he tells me. 'I get it.' And every possible variation of that thought. He doesn't push me, even when an evil part of my brain wonders if I want him to try. He either inspires me to fuck or he leaves me alone, and when he leaves me I try so hard not to breathe a sigh of relief. Now I can go to sleep, or get back to work, or do one of the many millions of things that are racing around my brain and pushing all thoughts of sex away. I try to look disappointed, while he smiles and tries not to.

Eventually, he stops trying altogether. We get into bed and he plays with his iPhone – occasionally wanking when he thinks I'm asleep. And I listen to the sound, feel the bed shaking gently and I want to scream at how unfair it is that I don't even want to join in.

Sex doesn't have to die, it really doesn't. No one confiscates your libido when you fall in love, but if that's the case then why won't mine work? What's wrong with me?

What's wrong with *this*?

Maybe It's OK To Say 'I'm Fine' Even When You're Not

(xojane.com)

Him: I spy with my little eye something beginning with 'P'.
Me: Is it 'precious minutes of my life being wasted on this game'?
Him: This is why we don't let you play.

I tell true stories. Beyond the myriad minor details that the brain will blur with time ('Did he really tell me to "get on his cock" or was the line something clumsier – less perfectly suited to this porn story?' 'How did that particular guy smell? I feel like I can remember it vividly, but perhaps I've just pieced it together from more recent memories of Mark'), everything's true to the best of my knowledge. But that doesn't mean it's honest: I lie by omission.

Commenters often think that the stories I tell are the sum total of the potentially embarrassing or kinky elements of my life. Well-meaning strangers say 'Oh, I love your honesty', and I wish I was even half as honest as they think I am. I'll explore the fuck-ups, sure, but only when they're funny. I once gave a gentleman an enthusiastic blow job in an alleyway, only to wonder afterwards why there was a horrible smell following me. When I reached the train station and discovered that my bag was covered in dog shit, I was utterly mortified. Did he know? Could he, while he fucked my mouth eagerly, see my bag in the background, sitting in a pile of something that'd come back to haunt me later? It took me a year to stop feeling those dark waves of pain rushing through my chest: the shame and the humiliation of it. When I had, though, I blogged about it, because exposure equals clicks. Or, to sound less mercenary, I'm happy to lay myself bare if it makes someone else feel better about the embarrassing things that have happened to them. If I tell stories about falling off the bed, chipping someone's tooth, or getting covered in dog crap during a seedy alleyway blow job, one reader may feel slightly better about that time they shit themselves during anal.

The alleyway event happened, by the way: as I say – I tell true stories. Then people think, because I reveal quite a lot, I must be telling them everything. But if the 'you're so honest' reaction is anything to go by, then the best spies of all will be the ones who tell you *almost* all of their secrets – hiding the genuinely private ones in a web of those that are superficially shocking. If you say nothing people prod you to open up, going crazy for the tiny scraps of info they can prise out of you. If you tell people *almost* everything you get away with some whopping lies by omission.

The loss of my mojo is one of those lies. I didn't tell the blog whenever Mark and I had yet another night of frustration, during which I'd cling to the duvet and try not to sob because my useless body wouldn't let me fuck. The other lies sit in the same ballpark. They're zipped up in my skin, and sometimes dotted and scarred across it. Sometimes growing out of it like the thick black hairs that I pluck from my collarbone. Nipples. Neck.

I don't tell people that I hate my body.

In a rare break in the panic and sadness, long after that terrifyingly suburban Wednesday, Mark and I are sitting in the garden on a picnic bench, sharing a joint and smiling at the world. It's sunny, which I hate, but we're at home, which I love, and Mark's idly fondling one of my legs and staring at the floor when he hits me with the weirdest declaration.

'They're pretty good, my feet, aren't they?'

His feet – a bit gnarled and a slightly odd shape, with those hard skin, yellow hoof bits on the sections that rub in his shoes. His toenails, wonky and thick and weird-looking, like basically all toenails are.

'Your feet?'

'Yeah. I mean, they're OK aren't they?'

'Sure. They're just your feet: they're normal feet. What made you say that?'

'It just occurred to me.'

The powerfully casual way he said it made me realise: I fucking *hate* my feet. I'd never hated them until that moment. I'd assumed they were just normal-ish feet. Same as Mark's, they have that hard skin in places and a couple of blisters and a dark line where the gunk from my flip flops has rubbed off. The nail varnish is chipped and the nails are too long and until this minute I hadn't noticed, because I'd been too busy concentrating on the rest of my body. I couldn't comprehend the ease with which he'd praise his own. Not just that he'd have the confidence to say it, when his feet are anything but remarkable: the very fact that he could feel that way at all. That there'd be an individual existing on this planet earth who did not hate every inch of their own flesh in every tiny grisly detail.

I've mentioned before that I write blog posts about how we should all love our bodies: how we should celebrate these miraculous vehicles that get us from cradle to grave, agony to ecstasy. Yet with every day that goes past I hate my body more. From the top of my dry, damaged hair to the tip of my chipped toenail varnish, and every ounce of fat and ingrowing hair and stretch mark in between. The only thing I hate more than my body is the part of my brain that *makes* me hate my body. The bit that's sucked up false ideals like a sponge, yet sits behind a hypocritical declaration that all bodies are beautiful, whispering in the background 'except yours'.

Because the worst kind of lie is the aspirational one I tell every day, when I explain to people that everyone is fine, and lovely and beautiful. I say it over and over to try and make myself believe it. Then I retreat to the bathroom to spread hair removal cream over every inch of my skin: stomach, thighs, chest, neck. Collarbone. Crotch. Toes. The more you look for it the more you find: those dark hairs that are gone one day and long the next. I have polycystic ovaries, and the ovary part doesn't bother me. The 'cystic' part doesn't bother me, as long as I try hard not to think about tiny spots growing inside of me, covering wet organs with a layer of pustules and... sorry. But something about having polycystic ovaries (PCOS, if you're a doctor, or you want to

Google it for kicks) gives me hormones. Or suppresses my hormones. Or makes me absorb too many hormones. To be honest, I wasn't listening to the science part; I was too busy praying for a pill. Each time I go to the doctor they say 'Oh lots of women get it', and 'It's not life-threatening', and the words go in one ear and out the other because all I want to hear is 'We can fix it'. They can't, by the way. They can give you advice and pills and they can try different things, but eventually you're stuck with the knowledge that you'll always grow hair on your neck. That the day you finish paying off your credit card debt for laser hair removal is the day you'll discover a fresh crop's just grown through. And you'll weep because it shouldn't matter, and because you're beautiful no matter what. And you'll feel, deep down, like that's a lie.

I don't really think it's a lie: I do think people can be beautiful no matter where they happen to sprout hair. But there's a big difference between knowing something rationally and believing it.

So I write blog posts to make other people feel better about themselves. And I vaguely hint that 'I'm quite hairy for a girl', and I pray they're imagining a political statement bikini line rather than the miserable truth of plucking hairs from my neck and nipples. Other women get this too. A good friend of mine plucks hairs from her neck in front of me – sitting in a field at a festival she gets the tweezers out and says 'god there are more of them each year', and I'm bowled over with shock and admiration. How has she managed to deal with this when I can barely speak the words out loud? I'm supposed to be the one who doesn't give a fuck. Look at me, caring, like a twat.

Like the warnings on cigarette packets, the fact that most pictures are Photoshopped is now common knowledge. So we're all expected to roar with confidence and ignore the nagging voices in our head that tell us we're no good. Women have it harder, because for so long our bodies have been considered open property – from website sidebars that cackle about our cellulite to men who tell us to smile in the street. 'Cheer up, love,' they say, as if they own the place, and the women are their customisable decorations. But while we've had it harder than men, they get it too. Mark thinks his feet are alright, but he's also been told to man up, be more muscular, grow a fashionable beard. Now shave the fashionable beard off because they're all a bit hipster now. I'm told to be 'beach body ready' and he gets a more playful 'Eat fewer pies'. The underlying assumption is the same: your value comes not from how you feel but how you *look*. Moving beyond that – as we are, slowly – the message becomes 'own your body' and 'love yourself', and it's better by a margin. It's the one I shout from angry blog pages. But I can't claim that message is 'honest', because it's never the full story. The whole truth requires that crucial caveat: 'We know it's hard. It's hard for everyone'. The omitted lie sits in the background, and I very rarely mention it: I'm not saying 'love yourself' to try and persuade you, I'm trying to convince *myself*.

When I hint at this stuff to Mark, he helps: as he always bloody does. He listens and calms, and strokes the back of my head like I'm a temporarily startled horse, and says, 'They know – everyone knows this is hard.' His lilting, resolute insistence that everything will be 'fine' is as constant as the sun rising tomorrow: it'll pass. Come lie in a darkened room with me and cry on my chest for a while and everything –

everything – will be OK. I don't think it will, but I omit that bit too, because I haven't the time to discuss it.

Someone's telling me something and I need to concentrate. It's about work: it's important. I can hear from the tone of their voice. But for some reason the words don't really come through. It's the Monday morning stand-up meeting: peppy Company X employees gather around in a circle competing to see who can be most impressive this week.

'We're launching our campaign today. Six months of work! We're hoping it'll go...'

Don't say 'viral', don't say 'viral'...

'...viral.'

Sigh. That was my job: to 'make it go viral'. But it doesn't really work like that and when you try to explain people think you're lazy. You can get up at six in the morning to plan and you can push for senior management to let you do a 'funny' video (the corporate definition of 'funny' being, of course, *not* funny), and if the worst comes to the worst you can shove thousands of pounds of budget behind a project, and still the best you might get is a half-hearted retweet of support. In the meantime, you'll be side-eyeing your phone to make sure it's locked, and hoping against hope that the sleep deprivation hasn't led you to do something stupid. You'll be answering to two names and online at all hours to make sure that everything gets enough clicks.

Something's definitely wrong. This job that I loved has become terrifying. I sit in the office, chatting to my colleagues through a fuzzy haze of panic and occasionally realise that I've done nothing for an hour: I've been staring at a computer and willing myself to send an email. Muscles so tense my arms are shaking. At the end of the day I'll zip through the station like a proper Londoner: dodging tourists and wheelie suitcases and drunk suits weaving from platform to platform. I glide through it and for a minute I feel good: I'm efficient and I'm getting things done. In my head I'm composing that email that I was too scared to send earlier: 'Apologies to senior management but I'm afraid this isn't possible', simultaneously working out what to post about later tonight 'I've a story from a while ago about the first time I pegged a guy with a strap-on'. And the disconnect doesn't feel weird when I'm stamping through the station, because that busy, efficient ball of panic is me: it's what I do. I run through stations juggling a phone, a kindle, a book, and notes scribbled frantically during that morning meeting. When I sit on the train I get back to work, and ignore the fact that my eyes feel funny. When I get home I vomit and it feels good, because that's what busy people do. They vomit and then wipe their mouths and get on with things.

The next day, my boss calls me to one side. We love my boss: she's efficient, smart and she gets things fucking *done*. She never pries into your personal life, but she'll understand if you tell her that you need a day off. She'll ask if it's an emergency but never what that emergency is. She's subtly warm: having learnt to pile efficiency on top of emotions to avoid all the labels that we otherwise give to women. Emotional. Caring. Likely-to-go-off-on-maternity-leave.

So when she makes the kind of sympathetic face my mum makes, I'm instantly worried.

'Is everything OK?'

My heart hammers: did she find out? Did I fuck up? Have I accidentally posted something on the wrong channel and a politician who should have been retweeting our campaign has ended up clicking on a post about butt sex? Or – worse – has one of the terrifying blog commenters, the ones who promise to find me... has one of them found me?

'I'm fine!' I tell her, slightly shrill but otherwise – I think – perfectly composed.

'You seem quite busy.'

'I am, yeah. There's a lot on.' And I smile. Because that's what you do – you smile. Then when she's satisfied that my smile isn't going to crack into a sobbing fit she wanders off.

And I run to the bathroom to vomit. Efficiently. Back at my desk within two minutes, I congratulate myself on a record.

Occasionally there's a break in the haze and I remember to chill out. These days I feel strange, heightened as if I'm ever-so-slightly stoned. Lucy, my married friend, who's now excitedly pregnant, is throwing a party to celebrate, and I throw out everything on my to-do list to make space for a visit. Except really I don't, because on the train I'm writing emails and I'm inviting Claire, because she's been asking to see me and I don't realise that 'killing two birds with one stone' is not an appropriate metaphor for having friends.

Lucy's the perfect person to visit when you're stressed, though, because everything around her exists in a state of cheery chaos. When I arrive for her casual 'we're pregnant so it's a great excuse for cake' party (emphatically *not*, as they explain, a baby shower), Claire notes that morning sickness hasn't dulled her enthusiasm for up-cycling: the place is covered in hand-printed muslin cloths and tiny bootees made from faded jersey fabric. It's not a bitch, it's genuine admiration – it'd be way too easy for me to toss out insults about smug, yummy friends who invite you to baby showers so they can show off how polished and neat their lives are. Lucy, however, maintains a healthy air of disorder. She never looks down at you, she's mostly looking at you over her shoulder through a blurry field of jam and scruffy hair, while she whisks frantically and tries to avoid knocking things over. Lucy would never have a real baby shower, because she wouldn't want people to feel they should shower her with things. She just has 'parties', at which random friends are invited to turn up 'at some point on Saturday' to eat sticky-iced cupcakes and alternate cups of tea with fizzy wine. Through the buzz of the party, Lucy asks if I'm OK, and it's an odd question: I *am* OK, but I've only just realised how not-OK I've been for quite a while. It feels like I'm on holiday from myself, so I make the most of it by gossiping with people, and making straight-faced suggestions for awful baby names.

Claire's divorce is just coming through, so naturally she's in the mood for a party. Unlike more judgy married friends, Lucy won't do that pursed lips thing, or ask Claire why the 'sudden' change of heart about her ex. Claire isn't yet sure how she feels about the compliment 'you look too young to be divorced!', so she spins the stories of recent Tinder dates, and we don't talk about the sad bits.

Claire and Mr Wrong had been together since they were young and this fun, funny, adorable guy seemed pretty much perfect for her. They bought a house together the year before they married, and I occasionally ventured all the way out of London to visit them. They had a great couple double-act – he'd cook, she'd pour drinks, he'd make a joke, she'd throw back the punchline before you even saw it coming. Later in the evening he'd break up any serious gossip by launching into ridiculous dance routines, or slurring excitedly about their local nightclub and how we should all pop down there before bedtime for a round of shots. From that perspective, they looked like one of those couples I'd always wanted to be – drinking wine together round the piano and verbally sparring until it was time to go to bed. As Claire patiently explained to me, though, it takes more than jokes and tequila to make a marriage. When they were alone their routine faltered. She'd still pour the drinks and he'd still cook, but in separate rooms, and without a laughing audience there was a howling silence to fill. The bustle of wedding preparation had occupied it for a while – the intricate planning and detail felt like Claire's version of Lucy's crafting: a shared hobby that excited them both. But as she walked down the aisle, Claire realised there'd been so many conversations about wedding favours, guest lists and venues that she'd forgotten how to talk to her husband about anything else. When they fired up the conversation again, neither of them had much to say, and the periods of silence grew. The loneliness grew. And to make things much, much worse, Claire was the only one who noticed.

By the end of the definitely-not-a-baby-shower, Claire and I are definitely-not-pissed, and we wobble together to the train station, trying to outdo each other in insistence that this wasn't really a proper night out. Lucy's pregnant, so it was very tame: far less excitement than we're used to. It wasn't, of course, but it makes us feel younger to pretend that there's more fun round the corner.

I sleep for most of Sunday, trying to avoid the panic that's rising in anticipation of Monday morning.

Later that week, we go out for dinner: Mark, Claire, Dave, my sister, me, a whole bunch of other people. I can't remember why – perhaps at Dave's suggestion ('One day we'll all be dead. Drinks?'), or maybe it's someone's birthday, or we're just celebrating the fact that we're reasonably young and fairly solvent and none of us have kids yet so we can. We get sloppy on cheap wine and eat Greek food, and Claire has us all in stitches with the latest instalment in her Tinder tales. My sister and I fight over who owes who money, and when I'm in the toilet she sneaks £20 into my wallet. By the time the bill comes I don't feel sick any more: I feel fine.

'How are you?' Claire asks. 'Better?'

'I… didn't realise I had anything to get better *from*,' I reply, and she gives me a quizzical look. I realise that other people have stopped talking, and a couple of them are joking about the way I got so heated over the money. In my slightly panicky way, I'd raised my voice as I realised that my sister wouldn't let me pay her back, and a couple of people in the room had looked over. Claire gives me a look that's a cross between worry and mockery – if she made a joke now I'd probably be OK. I could laugh and it would all be fine, and we'd go home happy after a good night out. But for better or worse, she doesn't. She hugs me, so I sob, and if she weren't holding me up I don't think I'd stay standing.

On the train on the way home, Mark frowns.

'Why,' he says 'do you have to be so weird?'

That's it – dead flat. No 'dickhead' or 'twat' or 'you bellend' to temper the question. He's not joking, but he's not angry either, he just doesn't understand what's going on. For months I've been twitchy about sex and more recently I've been rushing home after work, locking myself in the spare room and typing until I'm too exhausted to do anything but cry. I've always been occasionally 'weird', when I get an idea in my head that I've upset someone and I go full-on Mother Theresa trying to make it up to them, but now I'm struggling not to cry and spitting apologies before I even know what it was I did. After months of patiently accepting it and offering help that's swifty rejected, Mark finally asks me what the problem actually is.

'Why do you have to be so weird?' Again. Looking at me with an expression I rarely see: genuine frustration and hurt. At the time, it's just too much. I want to put the weird in a box and put my head on his shoulder, and feel his breath hot down the back of my neck and his eyes on my cleavage. Simple, easy, un-weird things.

'I just didn't want her to feel she should pay for me. No one should ever have to pay for me.'

'She wasn't paying for you.'

'I couldn't remember.'

'You weren't listening. You just freaked out and ran to the toilet.'

'I needed the toilet.'

'You were crying.'

'Was I?'

'Yes.'

'The bill thing mattered to me.'

'Well, it doesn't matter.'

Everything, I try to explain to him *matters*.

But at that point the only thing that matters is that we're having this fight – we're sitting on a train and instead of staring down my top or gripping my thighs he's looking directly at me, as if he's waiting for the tears to flow. As if the moment the tears start flowing is the moment he'll have proof of the 'weird' thing, which scares me because I don't want to be weird. Above all I don't have time to work out why I am, or how to stop. I hold the tears in.

I'm not weak. I'm fighty. I'll shout and get angry about things all the time. I have opinions on the Internet, for god's sake. I am used to people being pissed off with me. Buggered if I'm going to cry just because my boyfriend is trying to push me to explain why I cried in a restaurant, and why all my friends have started tiptoeing around me, as if just one wrong word will turn me to dust. I'm not weak. Besides, I don't have time for this bullshit: I have work to do and things to write and people to email and tweets to reply to, and even as he stares at me, waiting for an answer, my phone buzzes twice in my pocket.

'What's weird about being busy? What's weird about *caring* about stuff?' I'm trying to explain to him, in a way that keeps me on the moral high ground, just why I'm right. What's wrong with everyone else in the world that they're not always this busy too? How do they get through their lives without having a quick, nervous vomit before lunchtime and a nice long worry before bed?

'There's nothing wrong with being busy,' Mark explains as he puts his key in the front door and stamps inside. 'But you're more than that. You're... I can't think of the word.'

There *is* a word for it and I feel like if I can just get a bit more air to breathe I'll remember what it is. I step inside and collapse on the sofa, in a state that's even weirder. Wheezing like I'm ripping the air out of the room, unable to get enough in my lungs. All my limbs tingle and it feels like I might faint, but I'm safe here on the sofa with Mark looking over me. I don't look up, but I know the expression he's wearing: etched with worry and searching for the right words to stop me doing this... thing. It looks like a fit, but it isn't. I'm shaking and rocking and sobbing and wheezing but it's *not* a fit because I know that I could stop, I just need to try. If I could grow up for a second, and sort myself out, I'd be fine. Pull myself together.

There's probably something wrong with being like this: everyone's busy but maybe not everyone sobs in a tingling, shaking ball on the sofa while their boyfriend stands over them trying to think of a better word than 'weird'. I look back at some of the other things, struggling to work out which of them is normal and which the mistake. The jittery way I'll check my phone every five minutes. The searing flash of rage if someone delays me for two seconds at an escalator. The guilt if I don't reply to an email as soon as I get it. The permanent fear of being fired. Late nights spent trembling into my pillow as my brain flicks through endless to-do lists and impossible deadlines. The rushing sensation when, standing on a platform as the tube approaches, it looks easier to fall under than get onto it.

Is Your Mental Health Affecting Your Sex Life?

(*madlyinlove.org.uk*)

- Watching the bit where they bring out the wedding cake on Don't Tell The Bride *-*
Me: You know, maybe we should get married.
Him: Do you just want me to get you some cake?
Me: …yes please.

We're getting better at talking about mental health – charities and well-meaning celebrities are going out of their way to remove the stigma. But most people are still a bit wary of discussing it – as if saying 'I'm a bit fucked in the head' will paint you as a headfuck forever: a failure.

I thought exactly the same. There couldn't possibly be anything wrong with me: I'm normal, just busy: this is what busy people do. Maybe part of the reason we're rubbish with mental health is because we can never see inside anyone else's head. We can try and empathise, so when a friend tells me she's had a really depressing weekend I can think 'Sure, I know what that feels like. I've had pretty shit weekends myself.' But without the ability to sit inside her skin, feel the weight and the darkness of it, I don't know that my 'depressing' is someone else's 'No, actually I feel like I want to die'.

I don't have depression, by the way, that's not my thing. My thing – the word I was struggling for to replace Mark's 'weird' – is anxious. I have anxiety and until recently I thought everyone else did too. That the people I passed in the station were feeling the same way I was: that guy over there with the twatty Bluetooth headset and the shiny suit (estate agent or recruitment consultant, you mark my words) had the same constantly hammering heart, combined with a low-level ache in the pit of his stomach that he monitored when there was no bathroom nearby. Am I going to throw up? What if I get another email asking me to work late? Can I guarantee I'll get to the toilet in time? If you break your leg it's obvious to everyone, including you. It's a sudden, sickly snap. Everyone knows: they sign your cast and tell you to get well soon. But this thing happened so gradually I assumed it was just part of getting older. I'm a grown-up now, so of *course* I'll panic: I have so much more to panic *about*. Not getting all the housework done. Not hitting that deadline. Getting fired because of a stupid mistake. That mortgage application? Confusing, complicated, and has to be done today, so it's prime panicking material, ergo it's perfectly normal to spend an hour staring at the ceiling gulping air, and praying that Mark doesn't come home before I've pulled myself together. Those awful moments when Mark *does* get home before I've pulled myself together.

Shit, Mark. Have I fucked this up?

The last few months haven't just been unsexy – they've been lonely. That feeling of going to bed together, yet still being utterly alone, as one of you reaches out and the other holds their breath, trying to fight the desire to push them away. If Mark had been a bit less understanding, maybe I'd have spoken up earlier. But keeping things quiet is much easier to do if you're with someone who's so laid back he's horizontal most of the time. I think I wanted him to fight me but all he said was:

'No worries, I understand.'

I'd bite my tongue because apologies made things sound worse – like it wasn't fine at all. And they'd build until I'd want to scream them, so when I'd eventually let loose they'd come out with other, harsher words as company:

'You don't understand.'

'*How* could you understand?'

'Why are you so fucking *chilled* about everything?' The subtext, of course, is that if I see my worries as normal, then his calm is the total opposite. 'Why, Mark, are you so fucking *inhuman*?'

If he thinks I'm weird, then I think worse: at the height of my anxiety I think he's a borderline robot. Like that Rudyard fucking Kipling poem: triumph and disaster greeted with the same semi-shrug. The baffling belief that the world will keep turning even if we don't get this paperwork done on time. I never stopped loving him, but at my most vulnerable, I hated his chilled-out, cuddles-cure-everything attitude. That he could be so happy when I was running rings around myself and sometimes literally tearing at my hair meant every time I looked at him I saw someone to blame.

'Hey,' he'd say, coming up behind me and wrapping his arms around my waist. One of the hugs that he'd taught me to treasure felt suddenly cloying. 'Why don't you rest for a bit? We can sit on the sofa, play *Fable 3*, and I'll get you some wine.'

'No.'

'Gin?'

'No. You don't understand.'

He'd look at me with this weird, sad face and I'd get a kick of rage deep in my gut. After all, the reason I couldn't sit down and relax now was surely partly his fault: on top of the work-related list in my head there's a home-related list, that covers the housework and paperwork and life admin that seems to fall naturally on my shoulders instead of his.

What I should have done, of course, was tell him. Say 'Hey mate, how about you pick up a fucking dishcloth every once in a while if you want to be supportive?' But I didn't. I bubbled and simmered and added these extra things to my to-do list, then when he got upset and distant I'd add *him* to the 'to-do' list too. Next task: play *Fable 3* with Mark. Cheer him up a bit. Paint on a smile and muster some jokes. If I can multitask well enough maybe I can let him take the controller for a second, so I can keep one eye on the screen and another on my laptop, writing something for a 9am deadline. Drink the wine, too, to prove I'm still me, just need to make sure I don't get too sloppy. A glass, or two, or three or OK fine the bottle.

Somewhere along the line, around the time he got added to the 'to-do' list, Mark started to look like an enemy. Along with most of my friends, my family and anyone who wanted a slice of my time. Not the kind of enemy you physically fight, but a challenge you feel you should tackle. Tasks like 'go to the pub with Claire' and 'fuck Mark' are things that a sane, happy me would be itching to do, but as soon as they're added to the list they become a struggle. A friendly text from Lucy made the bile rise in my throat, as I choked down the desire to tell everyone to fuck off. Leave me alone. Stop *stealing my precious time*. As the tasks piled higher it was harder to remember which of them I used to enjoy, so instead of being a delicious relief at the end of a hard day, sex became a chore: yet another thing to tick off a destructively obsessive list. So I stopped seeing Claire, Lucy, Dave – everyone. I couldn't stop seeing Mark because he was always there at home, with his hugs and his worried face and his enduring, inexplicable love. So I stopped fucking him, I stopped hugging him and we barely touched from the jolt of the alarm in the morning until I pushed away his affection at night. The filthy porn fantasies about him in my head were replaced with a 24-hour audio track that tick-tick-ticked the seconds away until my next wobbling breakdown.

When you have someone who's given you so much happiness, it's hard not to blame them when that happiness disappears.

'What's up?'

'I'm sad.'

'Why?'

I don't know. I just literally don't know. But the more you care about it, the harder I'm going to try to find a reason that you can fix. If I'm stressed and you want to help, then I'll point to things you can do. Deliciously concrete things. Do the laundry. Wash the dishes. Get me a bottle of wine from the shop and don't raise your eyebrows when the whole thing's gone in an hour. Stop touching me. Stop loving me.

Just go.

See, this is why it's good to talk about sex: and of all the hypocritical failures I've made when I say one thing as GOTN and do the opposite in real life, this one has to be the biggest. I genuinely believed that because I was 'Girl on the Net: angry sex blogger and incorrigible pervert' that was my role forever. Mark had gamely put up with my excitable lube-related experiments and tendency to analyse every dirty fuck we ever had, but I figured that was one of the things he loved about me. So when that disappeared, and this horny girl who didn't give a fuck was replaced by someone who shook and panicked and literally *couldn't* fuck, what I should have done is talked to him about it. Instead I dissembled frantically, making excuses to stave off the conversations that I didn't want to have.

Give me time, I explained, and I'll get better. I'm just busy. I'll be back to normal soon, where 'normal' equals some combination of confident and permanently horny. A caricature of an Internet sex kitten with none of the bad bits that exist in real life. When guys asked me 'Where are the pervy women?' a *truly* honest answer would have been: 'Right now? This one's crying in the bathroom'.

I'm lying in bed one morning: a work day. Mark rolls over to slip his hand around my chest, cradling me for five minutes before we both have to get up. Unthinkingly, I twitch. My muscles tense up as I worry that we'll have to have morning sex: my least favourite kind. If I manage to get wet (which will be a rare miracle) then the alarm will go off halfway through and I'll be stuck in the weird limbo of trying to decide whether to ignore it, thus ruining the fuck with that nagging beep that reminds us we're late. Or I could reach over and turn it off, and risk spotting that I have 25 new emails: the gut-punch realisation that no matter how much time I have, the list will never be clear. Even if I could muster the energy for sex, the world would keep spinning even as we fucked. More tasks would pile up and the list would only get longer.

He buries his face in my neck and I feel his warm breath. His erection pokes me right where I used to love it – in the crack of my arse so I can feel it through my knickers. He lets out a gentle snore and I sigh with relief. Rubbing myself back into him so I can enjoy his body without the pain of worrying whether I'll have to do anything with it. But the tick-tick-tick of panic is still there, so I dare myself to get out of bed. This has become harder in the last few weeks, but so far I've managed to do it eventually, through sheer force of will and self-hatred.

'Get up,' I tell myself sternly. Like an angry gym instructor who's giving you more than your money's worth. 'Just move your legs and swing them out of the bed. Think of all the things you have to do! They're sitting in your inbox right now, calling to you. The people who've sent them will be getting angry. You'll be missing out on opportunities! You need to pull yourself together, you useless bitch. Go on – one leg. Just swing one leg out of the bed. Other people do this every single day. What's wrong with you? Do it.'

I lie there for another five minutes, wondering why I can't. It seems physically easy – I can conceive of doing it today as I did yesterday. What's stopping me is certainly not tiredness: I'm wide awake, sweaty, with my pulse racing, as if I've just finished a sprint and hopped into bed to recover. All I can think about is the list of things that awaits me when I look at my phone and suddenly the act of standing up seems impossible. While I'm here on this cotton-sheet island I'm safe, but as soon as I get out of it the mountain of tasks will topple down onto me.

'You are pathetic,' I tell myself. 'Grow up. Sort yourself out.'

This happens every morning for a week. For two days I'm late for work (arrive at work: vomit) and the next two I work from home (every couple of hours: vomit). On Friday I go to the doctor.

When I say it aloud it sounds a comically easy solution to this whole pathetic mess. You just went to the doctor? That's not dramatic – that isn't *plot,* it's just hypochondria. Again, though, it's another lie of omission. I'll agree with everyone on the Internet who tells me mental health is important. I'll shout from the rooftops about how mental illness is often misunderstood and we should treat it more like physical illness. People who tell depressed individuals to 'cheer up' or 'pull yourself together' – these people get hefty doses of my scorn and ire. Yet with mental health as with the body confidence thing, when it comes to myself, I can't conceive of things in the same way. Pride in your own body is for other people: because no one's body can be as gross as my own. Likewise support for mental health problems is for other people. I'm not sick enough for help; they need it more than I do. I just need to... pull myself together.

Because of this, I'm expecting her to throw me out in minutes, with a prescription for something placebo and a hint about wasting her time. But she doesn't – she sits patiently and wears the same confused face as Mark does.

'What would you like me to do?' she asks, holding out a box of tissues and hovering near her prescription pad.

'I don't know,' I tell her. 'I just want you to make it so I don't feel like this any more.'

She bites her lip and says, 'Hmm', and that in itself is a comfort. I like that she's uncertain: that the answer is no clearer to her than it is to me. Sharing the confusion feels like a minor success, and I blow my nose for the 25th time while she starts listing options.

'I could prescribe you something. But I'm not sure that's what you want. I could sign you off work. I could refer you to someone to talk to. The problem with the last one is that you'll have to go to sessions – you'll have another task on your list.'

'Yes! Exactly!' I nod and try to smile and I get that she understands. I'm not actually ill; I just need a rest. I'm like one of those Victorian ladies who fainted because she had too many society invitations, and all she needs is a week in bed with servants bringing her hot soup and she'll be right as rain again. The problem isn't with me: it's with the world. I explain part of this to the doctor, and she shakes her head.

'No, not that easy.' She's very firm, but she leans forward to soften the blow, making that sympathetic Mark-like face. 'You *are* ill, you know.'

'I am?'

'Yes.'

That's it. Just a simple, no-nonsense 'Yes'.

I'm ill. And as soon as she says it I feel a weight lift from my shoulders. The voice in my head has to shut up for a while, because I have her *permission* to be ill.

I try it on for size: 'I'm ill... But there's still loads to do. There's work and writing and...'

'I'll sign you off for two weeks. If I just do one they'll save the work for you to do when you get back. People take two weeks more seriously,' she explains. 'I can't make you better right now, but take two weeks to work out how you'd feel about the other options.'

She hands me a number and I fold it into the pages of a report that I no longer have to read and I feel light and fuzzy. As I leave the surgery it starts pouring with rain, and the rain feels so fucking *good*.

I'm not fixed – I'm not even *close* to fixed. But the word 'ill' acts like a safe word, giving me permission to stop without ruining everything. Stop doing things: sex, work, anything that makes you breathe like this and collapse into a puddle on the floor. Take a break. Stop.

10 Ways To Spice Up Your Sex Life

(mensjournal.com)

Him: What's that you're drinking?
Me: Wine.
Him: What kind of wine?
Me: White wine.
Him: No, but what's it called?
Me: Friday wine.
Him: OK, no more for you.

Mark tiptoes into the bedroom 30 minutes after I've gone to bed. I can hear the swish as he pulls his belt out through the belt loops and takes off his T-shirt and trousers. He's trying to be quiet, but it's not because he doesn't want to wake me. I'm lying in bed, having assumed the position: the one that makes me look deliciously asleep, but which he knows I never really sleep in.

Lying on my stomach, one leg raised slightly, thighs parted and knickers tight against my crotch. As Mark has kindly explained in intense and shivering detail, it's best like this. One buttock firm and taut, the other relaxed – ready to wobble just right if he gives it a smack.

I breathe deeply, pretending to be asleep.

This time, though, I'm not dodging an opportunity: I want him to do that *thing* again. The one where he joins in the game: pretends I'm asleep too, then gets into bed beside me and touches himself. Quick, urgent shuffles that I can hear, from my position buried face-down in the pillow. Strong enough that I can feel the bed shake as he rubs his prick under the duvet and the cover of darkness.

Part way through, I want him to reach over and touch me. Like he needs something to push him over the edge to orgasm. He'll put one heavy hand out and grope around until he settles on the tautness of my arse. He'll squeeze, rub, and pull at my knickers, to build a firm picture of my arse in his mind: pushing the fabric into the crack then reaching beneath the silk to get that skin-to-skin contact. When he gets there, he'll run his hot fingers down to test the wetness of my crotch, give a little moan in the back of his throat:

Unngh.

Like that was all he wanted.

His groping will get more intense and perhaps he'll roll over onto his side, trying to press his cock into my buttocks, rubbing the slick head of it against me as his hand movements get more urgent. This is my cue. Two years ago there were two options: I'd either wake up and slide onto him or sleepily bat him away. The latter and he'd retire to the lounge, the former and he'd slip it in tightly, right up to the hilt, and empty himself deep inside me, letting out one more muffled groan before rolling over to sleep.

But nowadays I'm rarely asleep: just anxious, tired and worried that my cunt's not working. So I do the new, third option instead: the one that shows him exactly what I want. I make the noise myself: *Unngh*. A mumbled, muffled moan. A moan comprised of sadness and an intense, gut-wrenching sob of lust. The moan that wants him inside me but can't quite have him, so will settle for the next best thing.

When I moan, he goes harder: fist pumping against his dick, dick resting against my arse, slapping noises as he whacks me with each stroke. When he comes, his spunk paints warmth over the back of my silk knickers, and I reach down to touch it before I fall asleep.

So what's changed to turn an 'argh no' into 'unngh yes please'?

Talking about it, for a start. Actually sitting down and having a conversation and saying things I should have told him months ago:

'I'm struggling a bit with shagging at the moment.'

He rolls his eyes and says:

'I'd noticed, dickhead.' Reaching out and pulling me by the shoulder so I'm lying close to his chest. 'It doesn't matter, you know. I don't mind.'

And there's a pause before he realises that's not the kind white lie he thinks.

'OK, I *do* mind. I really want to fuck you.'

'Ta. I want to fuck you too. I just never seem to want to fuck you at the moment you want to fuck.'

'Hmm. OK. Well, what *do* you want?'

That's how we got to the sleep-wanking thing. I love the sleep-wanking thing. The filthy feeling that I'm being used, without worrying that my body will betray me. For a few minutes I can forget that he knows it's a game, and pretend I really *am* asleep: that in my dreams I'll register his greedy, greedy hands all over me. That he's powered by such an urgent need to fuck me that he can't restrain himself from at least touching.

Lube helps too, of course. It's not magic by any means – it's not like I smear it on my junk and become an all-powerful sex wizard – but it takes one thing off the list. That humiliating moment when he tries to push himself in and I screw up my eyes and will my crotch to do... something. The feeling that I am, quite literally, a useless cunt.

I guess some of the credit should go to therapy as well, in case it looks like I'm recommending a cure for anxiety that involves a large, cuddly Northern bloke who cures you with magic spunk. Once a week I sit in a room with a lady who walks me through my latest panic attack, and dissect the anatomy of it. When does it get worse? How long do they last? How do you feel?

She makes me write an excruciating journal.

9:25am. Problem: Want to die. Reason? Email from a friend, that I don't have time to reply to.

3:35pm. Problem: Can't move arms or legs. Staring into space like a complete prick when I should be going to a meeting. Reason? There'll be a guy in the meeting who I forgot to say 'Good morning' to once. Been avoiding him ever since.

5:45pm. Problem: On the tube. Breathing like an

asthmatic running a marathon. Lady comes over to ask if I'm OK and I cry. Reason? Fuck knows.

8:50pm. Problem: Punched self in leg. Reason? Twitter.

She asks which tweet made me so worried and it turns out to be something ridiculous: a throwaway remark in reply to a joke that could lead to nothing dramatic. There's no logic in the panic, so the diary is helpful, because I want to *feel* like a logical person. I want there to be reasons for things. If 'A' then 'B'. If [terrifying situation at work] then [vomiting in a toilet]. I enjoy being able to make the link, even if the links sound thoroughly, desperately mad. I go to group sessions too, during which we're all far too polite to mention the therapeutic appeal of that sympathetic Schadenfreude: the sighing internal satisfaction of 'I'm not as bad as him...' It sounds cruel, but it's true, and I imagine for each time I think 'thank Christ I'm not so and so', So and So is thinking 'Thank fuck I'm not *her*.' Group therapy is held in the kind of room I imagine AA meetings happen in ('Hi my name's Sarah and I'm a complete fuck-up'). We bond – all fuck-ups together. And apart from a rather awkward incident with some guided meditation ('Tell me honestly: how did you feel about the meditation?' 'It made me want to eat my own face.'), it feels like it's partly working.

Perhaps the other thing that helped is that I quit my job. Not an option open to everyone, so as far as health advice goes it's right up there with 'eat more overpriced avocados' as a bullshit solution. But it helped me. It turns out that if there's one thing in your life that causes most of your stress, stopping that thing is an excellent idea. By the time I went off the rails, my job had turned from a fun and exciting way to spend the middle of the week to a hellish nightmare of stress upon stress. I used to fantasise about ways to escape. Not the normal fantasies that we all daydream about: that impassioned exit speech you'll make to senior management in which they'll see the error of their ways and promote you to CEO, or where you idly wonder if you can set off a fire alarm without people noticing. No, I mean genuinely weird things like making plans to break a leg, or contract a specific illness that would give me a couple of weeks in hospital. Nothing life-threatening, just enough that I could repeat the joy of that sign-off letter from the doctor, and feel like they'd be falling to bits as I loped off into the sunset.

I wasn't exactly the linchpin on which the entire company turned. No one individual ever is. And realising that was incredibly freeing. Anxiety often made me feel like any failure on my part would bring everyone tumbling down with me, so when I realised I wasn't that important I found it easier to work out what I wanted. If I don't rush to the office to arrive at 9 o'clock, who'll care? No one. Understanding that leaves me free to wonder whether *I* actually care. I don't.

Quitting my job gave me a bit of time to work out what I did want to do. I ran through the same question for other things in my life – who will care if I *don't* do this? If that particular blog post doesn't go live this instant, who will be upset? Well... me. Sex writing turned out to be one of the few things I was doing not because I had to, but because I *wanted* to. I had saved a bit of money that I could live on while I persuaded people to pay me to do it, so I could still hold on to the fragile pride that meant I couldn't ask for help from Mark. And hiding inside writing sounded like the best course of action, when getting on a tube made me sick.

Of course in order to write about sex, I had to get my mojo back and start *doing* it.

Mark picks up The Doxy and raises his eyebrows. 'It's fucking massive, mate.' And it is. A gigantic baseball bat of a sex toy, rather coyly referred to as a 'massager' but clearly designed for your genitals rather than your glutes. If you've heard of a Hitachi Magic Wand you'll have an idea what this one looks like. It's similar, only with a softer head, and far more power. If the Magic Wand is a supercar then this one's a fighter jet and in a world where I am struggling to enjoy the things I used to love, nuking the fuck out of my clitoris feels like a healthy step to take.

It's an awkward admission: that I want a sex toy to kick start me. Those sex tip articles where they talk about putting the spice back into your sex life have always turned me off, if only because the inclusion of novelty has never, for me, been something that ramps up my sex life – only something that enhances it when it's already going pretty damn well. In the past I've had threesomes, enemas, been to fetish clubs and bought love-eggs to pop inside me and see if they felt nice, but all these things were done while riding a wave of sexual enthusiasm. With no enthusiasm, will 'spicing things up' actually feel a bit more like 'scrabbling desperately'? After all, some of the best sex I've had with Mark has been, if not exactly vanilla, then at least fairly straightforward. In the door, rip each other's clothes off, fuck like rutting dogs, jizz ourselves: repeat. Surely if we're looking to rekindle a flame, the best way to start would be to do what we used to do when the fire was burning brightest? Not chuck new sex toys and positions at the problem, like a desperate salesman: throwing in a free badge, pen, £50 cashback bonus, whatever you like, just please for the love of god don't go.

Bringing new toys into the bedroom is, for me, a dangerous game. I love sex toys and there are a million and one things that I'll gleefully shove in me, on me, or up against me until I make the special face. But in a situation where I'm already feeling fragile and unsexy, the wrong thing could leave me feeling even weaker. Like I got dressed up to the nines for a special party and my date never showed up.

This toy, though? This one was interesting. Where I can't get excited about silky lingerie or romantic massage candles, a turbo-charged fuckwand that is powerful enough to make the walls shake? I can get behind (or under, or on top of) that. Even if it did nothing for my clit it'd give me a sense of satisfaction: the kind you'd get from riding a mechanical bull for a minute without being hurled to the ground. Worse case scenario, it was big enough that I could conceivably use it to defend myself against burglars.

Mark chooses to suspend judgement on it until we've plugged it in and fired it up.

His judgement remains suspended for about two seconds: the time it takes for the toy to kick-start into life with a deep, rumbling whirr, and for Mark to press it ever-so-gently onto my clit. About a second later I'm keening like a terrified banshee.

'Jjjgg kkkkfff.'

He looks at me in shock.

'Oh god, I'm sorry. That didn't work, did it?'

'Ngggg.'

I writhe in something which feels to me like ecstasy but looks to Mark quite remarkably like agony. He's flustered, and he pulls it away.

'Are you OK?' Struggling to summon the power of speech, I grab his hand and push it back onto my cunt, bringing the weird, delicious, rumbling new sensation with it.

'Put. It. Back.' Nervously, he does. For the next few minutes I wriggle, moan and bark weird groaning noises at the ceiling, screeching hideously if he moves it away from the magic spot for even a tenth of a second. He starts getting the tingles in his wrist that you get when you're sanding a wall. When I come, he stares at me with wide eyes and one of the hardest erections I've ever seen, declaring:

'You sound like a fucking lunatic.'

We give it a few minutes, to allow my clitoris a short respite before the next ecstatic assault, then begin again: this time recording my bizarre sex noises for posterity.

There's an old cliché that one of the hardest things to say to someone is 'please help me' and that's particularly true if you've built your life, and a fairly large chunk of your personality, on being someone who never needs help. When you do this too much, to a certain extent you condition your friends and family to stop offering. A simple, 'no thanks I'm fine' is soon replaced with 'no', which eventually becomes 'leave me the fuck alone', and before you know it you've trained most people around you to stop trying to help when you're struggling. Of course, as Mark points out, that means that the people who are nice enough to want to are left in the cold, wishing they could do something but too scared to battle my stubbornness, while the people I end up hanging out with are the ones who wouldn't notice if I burst into tears in a Tesco. Lucy would notice: she'd be juggling a baby in one arm and a handmade basket full of organic veg in the other, but she'd notice. She'd ask me if I was OK and she'd make that concerned face that people do when they're not sure how to react, but she'd ask. Claire would ask. Dave would ask. But ultimately none of them would ever see the true extent of my oddness: just the occasional few moments when things welled up hard and I couldn't quite keep them suppressed. Mark, on the other hand, saw all of it, and that's why I thought he would leave me.

It's easy to see your own mistakes and flaws as total deal-breakers. There's a lot of relationship advice that tells people to avoid certain behaviour – as if it's morally abhorrent. Depending on the kind of publication you're reading, these might be legitimate reasons for leaving (cheating, or abusive behaviour), or just hilariously sexist lists of things that are mildly annoying, such as not replacing the toilet roll or wiping your dick on the curtains. Because these things are so wildly different, it can sometimes be tricky to work out what actually counts as cause to end a relationship. When it's shit living inside your own head you eventually persuade yourself that no one else would want to deal with you either, and you trap yourself in a spiral of not asking for help, then refusing help, then wondering why the people who want to help you don't just leave you for someone more interesting. As Mark explains, though, you don't dump the love of your life just because they've gone on holiday for a while.

So what do you do? It's always tempting to offer a deluge of solutions: like a cheap clickbait list giving you Ten Ways To Fix Your Sex Life After You've Had A Breakdown. But truthfully, although I can tell you what helped me, I think the answers will be different for everyone. Mark threw a few suggestions of his own into the mix, offering me 'meditation' of his own invention: him squeezing me in a tight hug for 20 minutes or so while whispering 'Sssh' into my ear ('Was that better than the meditation in therapy?' 'Made me want to eat *your* face.' 'In a good way?' 'No.'). He teased me when I got stressed about things, which was hit and miss in just the right way – if you've spent six months throwing wobbly panics about anything from a missed train to a £1,000 overdraft, sometimes a bit of piss-taking helps you put things into perspective.

Alongside the odd experiments, the only thing that could count as a genuinely universal solution would be this one: talk. Talking can be hard if you've spent six months trying to keep your mouth shut in case it accidentally spits forth all the bizarre things you're trying not to think about, but luckily (or frustratingly, if you're also keen on the whole 'independence' thing) Mark had a solution for that too.

We sit in the living room surrounded by Post-it Notes. I have a glass of wine to hand, he has a cold can of Coke and we spend five minutes frantically scribbling things. I'm a bit worried that I'm not doing it right, as I realise I've just wasted thirty seconds of the time limit watching his sexy hands gripping the pencil, and wondering if he's thinking the same about me.

'Concentrate,' he tells me. 'Just think about what you've wanted to say over the last week.'

It's called a 'retrospective', apparently, and it's borrowed from his work, where programmers apply whatever magic logic they have to work out how to do things better than the rest of us. The idea is that, at the end of a software project (correction: at the end of each *stage* of a software project, because a project never truly ends and... sorry Mark I really don't get how this works at all) everyone chips in their thoughts on what went well, what went badly, and what they'd like to have done if they had more time. I'm used to this kind of thing from Company X, when we used traffic light colours to tell people about their work, although there it was simply a neat way to apportion blame. Euphemisms such as 'lessons learned' are usually code for 'get ready to bitch':

'In this project I learned the lesson that you need to give Jeremy from IT more time than usual to do anything because – oh haha no I'm obviously being light-hearted – he's a difficult cunt.'

Initially I roll my eyes and suggest that if we're going to borrow techniques from wanky online start-ups, perhaps we should go the whole hog and get a ping-pong table and a couple of pointless scooters as well. But after the first go I realise it's a neat trick. Mark's sneakily getting me to focus on the Post-it Notes, hoping the distraction will make it easier for us to talk without me bursting into tears halfway through. In this instance, the point of the exercise isn't to blame: like the coffee he lets me make him, the Post-it Notes are there more for me than him. As long as there's no animosity, and neither of you is really going to do the passive-aggressive 'lessons learned' thing, you can learn a shitload more about each other.

This is what we learned:

Me: that Mark hates it when I do the washing up ten minutes after I've asked him to do it.

Mark: that I am sick of washing up.

Mark: that I hate having to ask for lube, because it makes me feel like a failure.

Me: that he *likes* it when I ask for lube: that the very act of asking is, to him, a massive turn-on.

Mark: that I miss spanking.

Me: that he doesn't spank me because he's nervous. If he's not sure I'll enjoy sex at the moment, missionary vanilla sex seems like a better way to tempt me back into it.

Mark: that it's not.

And thus everything was magically fixed.

OK, not quite. But at least we had a better idea of how to start rekindling whatever we had before my being a mad fuck-up poured cold water on it. He was no more keen on Cosmo-style advice than I was and the idea of 'injecting the spice back into our relationship' sounded both painful and unnerving. What's more, he was firmly with me in the belief that we were pretty fucking spicy to start off with.

Over the course of the next few months, he patiently ran through the options we'd decided on: the sleep-wanking. Big tick. The Doxy: double-tick. Repeated application of vast quantities of lube: tick. Porn – a carefully curated combination of his filth and my less mainstream choices – played while we lounge on the sofa: tick. Soft kisses and gentle hugs and long sessions of foreplay: big cross. Worth a try, though, especially given that he's nervous about my reluctance. He has nightmares that one day he'll push me too far and I'll clam up completely, so the gentleness is a combination of tenderness and his genuine desire for something warmer. It's still not my thing, though. Flipping me over, holding his cock at the entrance to my cunt, and telling me I can't have it till I beg: tick. We mix and match for compromise.

We even tried the dirty-romantic hotel shag thing. No roses or Travelodge deals, just a cottage in the middle of nowhere and the kind of sex that made me remember why I loved it.

Like the kidnap scene which Simon staged for Mary, something about this fuck was so perfectly personal to me that it couldn't have done anything but hit the spot. You know when someone tries to dirty-talk you and it simply doesn't click? Whether they use a word you're not keen on ('pussy' – bleugh) or start describing an act that leaves you a bit cold, even just the tiniest misfire in what they say can be a greater turn-off than if they didn't speak at all. This shag was the opposite of that: a Mark-led monologue of words and phrases so hot that I still play them in my head today. So perfectly and instinctively tailored to me that every time I think of it I get the same lustful sensation as I had that afternoon – that kick in the gut. This feeling is far more visceral than heartache: it's a horny nostalgia – arousal tinged with the sadness that you'll never hear that phrase in the same way, for the first time, ever again. So memorable you get it like an earworm, which you can't evict until you lie in a darkened room and frig yourself cross-eyed as you conjure every detail of that moment.

Mark got out of the car and beckoned me to follow him. On the journey home we'd been touching each other – just gently. Teasingly. Hands and fingers stroking paths through the other one's clothes. His hand idly placed on my bare knee, pushing the hem of my skirt up further so he could grip the exposed flesh on my thigh. My fingertips stroking the tip of his cock through thin cotton trousers, idly wondering if I could cause that tell-tale spot of liquid in his crotch.

When we got out of the car he led me straight to the bedroom. No raised eyebrows, no questions – we marched straight in there. This in itself made me burst with happiness: there had been times when he'd been so gentle and reluctant that I worried I'd never see that determination again. He ordered me out of my clothes and I stripped. Told me to kneel on the edge of the bed and I did.

Each order was precise: put your face down into the bed. Lift your arse. Put your hands on your thighs and spread yourself wide. As I followed his instructions I could hear him behind me, undoing his belt and unzipping his trousers and the rustle as he pulled his dick out of his pants.

For the first time in a long time, I felt the trickle of wetness down my thigh. My cunt ached – that horny nostalgia reminding me that it hadn't hurt this hard since I was young and eager and bereft of a guy who was willing to come and fuck me.

When Mark pushed his cock inside me I let out what felt like a sigh of relief. All the times I'd said no, and all the moments when I'd sobbed myself to sleep feeling dry and useless and pathetic: they all came out in that breath.

Then he smacked me.

'Hold still,' he ordered, and the shivers came again. The pulsing waves in my cunt that responded so quickly to being told what to do. I held still.

He fucked me harder.

I moved.

He smacked me harder.

I moved one more time, deliberately – just a knee moving an inch or so to the left, enough to incur the faux-wrath that I knew would finish me off completely.

He hauled me back into position, his big hands moulding my body into the perfect shape: whether it was for visual appeal, or just the joy of having that power, or perhaps because having my legs at that angle made my cunt even tighter round his cock, I couldn't work out. But I didn't need to.

Because when he'd posed me into just the right position, he started fucking again. Quick, hard thrusts that spoke of his desperation to come hot and hard inside me. Just as I was aching and weak and tremblingly ready to come, he whacked me one more time, as a warning, and said:

'If you don't hold that position, and I can't come, I'm going to beat you *so hard*.'

No more omission: if I'm really honest sometimes the things that worked were totally unpredictable. A phrase, like that, for instance, which shot straight to the filthy kink centre of my brain and jolted it awake. I don't want to pretend I'm better; I'm just not as bad as I was, but we're making progress. It wasn't new positions or romantic breaks or a specific set of magic beans that did it: it could be a look from Mark that had me panting, or an outfit he wore that showed off the bulge of his shoulders and his tightly-packed junk in the crotch. There were no 'mind-blowing sex moves', just a lot of tiny moments that helped me remember what blew my mind about sex in the first place.

Live Your Life As If Everything Is A Miracle

(goodlifezen.com)

Me: Mary Poppins *or* Jurassic Park?
Him: Unless they've remastered Poppins and it now has a T-rex, that question is redundant.

'You just get to the stage where you can almost read the other one's mind,' the guy says, leaning across the table towards his girlfriend, who makes the necessary 'I'm going to be sick' face.

'See?' he slurs triumphantly. 'I knew she'd do that before she did it.'

Mark raises an eyebrow at me across the table. See, I know exactly what *he's* thinking too, and perhaps that in itself is a bit of a miracle, especially since we're pissed and it's three in the morning: it'd be a miracle if I could read an exit sign.

'Can you, though? You're not really mind-reading,' Mark explains, killing the romance with sexy science.

'You've just learned to read their behaviour. It's familiarity, not magic.'

'Well, sure. But it can be pretty intense sometimes. Like when I'm just thinking about ringing her and as I reach for the phone she'll call.'

He's wrong about the magic, obviously: no one can read someone else's mind any more than they can heal them with prayer, but let's roll with him for a second, because the romantic part of my brain wants to agree. I may not be able to guess a number Mark's thinking of, but there are any number of everyday things that feel to me like miracles. After a sarcastic back and forth, and another sip of our drinks, we establish a game and a set of rules.

'Paper, scissors, stone,' Mark offers. 'You both do it at the same time and let's see if you can match more than three in a row.'

She laughs and holds out her hand. 'We're going to be shit at this, but let's try.'

'Eyes closed?' asks the guy. A few other people look over to see if they manage it. I can tell some people are thinking what I'm thinking: how would *I* do with my other half? Absurdly, I have a competitive desire to see them fail, so that Mark and I can have a shot at trying three matches in a row. But I squash that feeling and instead start rooting for them. It's bollocks, after all, and the guy seems so keen to nail it. Perhaps the sheer strength of his desire to win will help them deliver a 3am miracle.

Let's look at some of the everyday miracles that Mark's performed for me. I know, an extraordinary claim requires extraordinary evidence – I'm not going to tell you he walked on water or anything, although he does frequently turn £10 notes into boxes of cheap wine. But in a world where most of us live in a vague fog of self-hatred, surrounded by media that tells us we're worthless, even the most basic acts of love can feel like magic.

So, miracle one. It was a shitty, rainy Saturday and Mark was doing something incomprehensible on his laptop – typing letters, numbers and brackets in a specific combination that would spit out an app of some kind. That's not the miracle, although it could be. Just as technology from the future would be indistinguishable from magic, so skills I lack strike me as miraculous. Can you recite the periodic table? Play guitar? Work out the bill split in a restaurant before the waiter returns with the card machine? You may as well be a wizard to me. Anyway, as I say, that's not it.

While Mark's working, he likes loud music: an electronic, drum-and-bass-y background dirge. To him it represents 'getting in the flow' but to me it sounds like an actual panic attack. I was teasing him about his music; in a way that I thought was playful.

'Could you turn it up a little bit? I don't think my eardrums are bleeding yet.'

'You're not...' Long pause while he loses his train of thought... '... funny.'

So I reach over to the stereo and turn it down ever so slightly. He doesn't notice. I do it again. He still doesn't notice. I try a third time and it becomes clear he's noticed, as he raises his eyebrows and – still staring at the screen – tells me that I should get on with my own work and leave him in peace for five minutes. He uses the tone he uses when he's joking, so I do it one more time.

'ARGH,' he shouts, as the music quietens to a whisper, 'why do you always have to be such a prick?

Usually fine, of course. In the language of love 'prick' means 'princess' and I should take it as a compliment. But the look on his face is now a blend of anger, hurt, and frustration. I can't actually read his mind, but if I could I imagine there'd be a screed in there about the fact that I don't take him seriously, and that I stomp over what he wants when I'm bored and want my way. He's right, and that hurts, so I take myself off to the bedroom and cry into the pillow for a while. It's great therapy: ask any teenage girl. That's not the miracle – that Mark managed to get a message through my own self-absorbed mind and pierce me in the cold lump where my heart used to be. No.

The miracle came the next day, when his key clicked in the lock and he came running through the hallway shouting my name.

'Ugh,' he grunted, as he pulled me into a hug. 'It's been a long day. I fucking *missed* you.'

I told you it wasn't magic: there's no water into wine or leper healing or any of that. But in the context of all the shit he takes from me, and the numerous times I hurt him, that he can walk in the front door after eight hours away, actually *missing me*? That's a miracle, right?

I still have a card on my mantelpiece that he gave me when he came home. Inside it reads: 'I'm sorry I called you a prick.' He thinks I keep it to prove I was right, but I don't. I keep it because I want to remember how I felt at the time: like him missing me was a genuine miracle.

Let's go back to paper, scissors, stone, and see how our couple got on. The answer is not bad. They did actually manage three matched pairs in a row. Double rock. Double rock again. Double paper. I made suitably impressed gasping faces, and a couple of people started a drumroll for round four. Can they do it? What are the chances? I can tell you now while I'm at a computer: the probability of winning three paper, scissors, stone games in a row is 1/27. The chance of four? Much lower: 1/81. It's not proof that they're mind-reading, but it'd be a fun end to the evening.

They fail, of course. On the fourth throw one goes scissors and the other sticks with paper. As if to redeem their telepathic connection, they simultaneously shout 'fuck it' when they open their eyes to see the result.

But, like a group of drunk twats who've got the bit between their teeth, we couldn't help but turn it into a competition.

Mark and I stepped up to the plate.

Mark's second everyday miracle is easier to explain.

'I saw a girl today on the tube.' Most of his girl-seeing happens on the tube, in part because he's not a reader. While everyone else skim-reads the 'Rush Hour Crush' section of the Metro he has a bit more time to people-watch. 'She was super-hot, and she reminded me of you...'

'Ah, thanks mate.'

'...because she had sideburns just like yours.'

Loud record-scratch.

'My *what*?'

'Your sideburns. Like, you know how your hair grows down further in front of your ears than it does with most girls? It's well sexy. Fancy a brew?'

And he turned round to pop the kettle on, as if it was *no big deal*. As if it was totally normal to take one of the myriad things I've always hated about my body and hold it up as 'sexy'. I stood in gobsmacked silence for a minute or two while he fiddled about with coffee cups and the interminable aluminium grinder.

'You think they're... sexy?'

'Yeah, of course.'

'Not... weird and gross?'

'No.'

And he opened the fridge to get the milk.

OK, so this isn't miraculous like a unicorn or anything, but if you could take pictures of normal horses and find that your shutter showed them to be white and glowing, with a single horn on their head, you'd certainly say that was pretty unusual. The hairy thing obviously bothers me, and you can't hide 'sideburns' the way you can hide a rogue nipple hair, so I try to pretend they aren't there. When you've spent your entire life believing that one feature is something you should either fix, hide, or steadfastly never mention, someone not only mentioning but *praising* it is a strangely lovely shock. There were no wands involved, but the glow of pride I felt when I looked into the mirror certainly felt like magic.

OK, back to the challenge. Could we manage more than three paper, scissors, stone matches in a row? I really wanted to win this, and I could see from Mark's sparkling eyes that he was aiming for the exact same thing.

We began with paper: a match. Half-hearted clapping ensued, which I felt was underselling it a bit: after all, the odds of two separate couples getting a match first time had to be pretty high – one in nine or something. We closed our eyes and tried again.

Double rock.

More clapping this time, we knew we'd done it before we even opened our eyes.

Again, eyes closed: double rock.

A cheer. A little bit of tension. Good-humoured tension, though, because we all knew it was arse: no amount of matches would make us believe in miracles. But we'd have loved to win just by sheer dumb luck.

One more? To beat the other couple?

Double. Fucking. Scissors.

I wanted to pick Mark up on my shoulders and carry him around the garden. He closed his eyes again – aiming for one more.

Double paper.

'Fuck off,' said the guy from the other couple. Quite fairly, I think.

Double rock.

Double paper.

We were on fire! Not reading each other's minds as such, just letting our hands do what felt natural. We sped up.

Double rock.

Double rock again.

Nine – we were up to nine! Nine motherfucking matches! The probability of that, I can tell you now that I have the Internet in front of me, is one in 19,683.

Not bad for two people who don't believe in magic.

But the human brain likes round numbers, so leaving it at nine would have seemed like a cop out. We needed ten. One more match.

To the soundtrack of other partygoers shouting 'You're fucking weird!' or 'Cheats!', we turned our backs to do the final one.

Double paper.

Jackpot.

The third miracle: Mark's still here. And I know, it's another of those ones where I cheat because no one actually waved a wand or did anything to break the laws of nature: that's why I'm telling you about them, though. When good things happen we often chalk them up to luck, or effort. Occasionally we don't notice them at all. But when he could easily have left, the fact that Mark's still here seems miraculous to me, and it feels like it deserves a prayer of thanks.

Still here after months of me sobbing for no reason, acting weird around our friends and cancelling events at the last minute; after endless soul-searching about my job and a final decision to leave it; that Mark expended infinite patience helping me find my sex drive again. There were countless nights holding me on the sofa, occasionally pinning my arms to my sides so I felt that tight, constricting comfort that helped me relax. Even when I disappeared for days and weekends, taking time away from him because I couldn't separate his love from my anxiety. After all the times I've hurt him, the gallons of forgiveness coffee, Mark's still here and he's kind enough to love me.

Just as we don't give ourselves enough credit for our own success, so we don't always give our loved ones credit for the tiny miracles they perform every day. When we feel low and shitty and worthless, and someone calls round or texts to ask: are you OK? Can I help? Nothing fell from the sky, there was no 'abracadabra', but if you feel better, that's enough of a miracle. Perhaps even *more* miraculous are those times when their support doesn't work, but they keep on doing it anyway, as Mark did: making dinner, distracting me with card games, sitting beside me for endless hours while I cried. Being there even when I didn't think I deserved company, or making himself scarce when I needed time alone.

I'm sorry I can't give you actual magic, but in a world where Mark is still here, after all of this bullshit, I reckon I can give you a miracle.

There are four explanations for what happened with the paper, scissors, stone thing.

One: it was a coincidence so huge that I am personally kicking myself for wasting that good luck on a crappy game. The probability of ten matches in a row, happening purely by chance, is one in roughly 59,000. Only slightly higher odds than matching five numbers in the lottery.

Two: it was genuinely miraculous, and love is so powerful it gives you telepathic superpowers. After so much time together, building empathy and understanding, Mark and I are now capable of literally reading each other's minds.

Three: the whole story is a lie. I'm so desperate for you to think Mark is cool that I'll break my primary rule and tell a whopping, deliberate lie to make him look like a borderline god. It's possible, and far more credible than explanations one and two. The only thing you'd need to work out is whether I made the *entire* story up, or grounded it in a little bit of truth. Perhaps the party challenge happened, and the first couple got three, but Mark and I only managed two matches before failing, then collapsing into a heap of giggles and bowing down to the reigning champs.

Four: the truth. This one goes back to the everyday romance that I mentioned before, when Mark and I counted pennies on New Year's Eve. In this version love isn't about lies or miracles, it's about the desire to spend time on otherwise boring tasks, for the sheer joy of doing them together. It's about giggling playfulness, and the ability to ignore your friends when they shout 'Cheat!' across the table. The fourth – and truthful – explanation started with a weird idea that we stuck with because it sounded like fun.

What I'm saying, I guess, is that Mark and I constructed a ten-step paper, scissors, stone routine, practised until we both knew it by heart, then waited nine months to perform it so we could trick our drunken mates.

How To Forgive Someone Who Has Wronged You

(lifehacker.com)

- Watching Anne Boleyn get beheaded on The Tudors *-*
Me: If I were getting beheaded, would
you come and watch?
Him: Depends. Are there snacks?

What's your type? Don't be coy; most of us have one, although it's usually hard to sum up in simple terms. Men are given a poor choice when it comes to describing their ideal fuck. Straight guys are asked if they're a 'tits' man or an 'ass' man. Gay dudes are encouraged to prefer twinks, otters, bears: shorthand codes for particular 'types', like smooth young guys, hairy dudes, big hairy blokes with chests you want to bury your face in. No matter which you prefer, none of the 'types' can come close to bottling that particular *je ne sais quois*. Straight women are usually encouraged to pick between celebrities: Brad Pitt or George

Clooney? Idris Elba or Daniel Craig? Team Edward or Team Jacob? Like there's a production line of blokes and you just have to select a few custom features to kit out the love of your life: suit or jeans? Beard or clean-shaven? Nerd or jock?

I could talk for hours on the kind of guy who's my 'type'. Skinny, emo-looking, wry-smiling guys with quick wit and slim wrists. Men who make jokes that aren't quite innuendo and laugh at mine in return. Who flash their eyes at me and curl their lip upwards, making me wonder if it's a sneer or an invitation. What they actually look like matters less than this devious, delicious aura of dirty sex. These are the kind of guys who'd cheat on their wives for a five-minute fumble in the toilets of a dirty Wetherspoons on the outskirts of town. They'd beat themselves up about it afterwards, but that wouldn't stop them thinking about it later, nursing an aching erection and wondering whether to call. But a guy could fit all these criteria and *still* not be one of them: my type, I mean. I'm neither Team Edward nor Team Jacob. I'm Team: 'both of them if they're up for it, ideally with a change of ends halfway through.' While I can see the hotness in most people, my 'type' is usually indefinable – I'll see him staring coyly at me over a pint and there'll be a stirring of interest. When I'm introduced, if he gives an oh-so-shy look at me, talks about his nerdy hobbies with just the right amount of self-deprecation, or simply has a look in his eyes that I can imagine he has when he's touching himself: I'll know. There'll be an electric fizz of temptation so powerful I'll feel like I should run away.

Because while I love the guys who are my type, they're dangerous.

Unfortunately, with the return of my mojo came a wave of temptation so strong it gnawed away at me, in the pit of my stomach and the back of my brain, whispering: you want to fuck *everyone*. The first was a guy I met briefly when I went to the pub with some friends.

'This is my partner,' a friend explained. She pointed me towards a guy who was leaning back nonchalantly in a chair, sipping something non-alcoholic and looking lithe and energetic enough that he might hop up any minute and go run round the block. Athletic isn't normally my thing, but 'my type' is never consistent, he can sneak up on me. With this guy it wasn't his body or face or hair (although a well-placed piercing and a decent tattoo certainly helped to nudge it along). It was something about the attitude. A simmering, confident sexuality beneath a surface-level nerdiness.

I said 'Hi', he said 'Hi' and we shook hands. My mouth said 'Nice to meet you' while my brain said 'Put your hand round my throat and squeeze tightly while you fuck me'. It's likely that this bloke thought I was odd, as I sat for the rest of the evening trying not to talk to him in case I stared too hard. Perhaps I look like I'm playing hard to get. If I'm really generous then I could say I'm being coy – aloof and mysterious. Actually I'm just incapable of having a conversation with someone sexy without dribbling wine down the front of my shirt.

He sipped his drink and I watched his slim hands curve around the glass. He leant back in his chair and I tried not to gawp at the thin sliver of skin peeking over the top of his jeans. When he grinned at me I smiled back, guardedly, as if the very act of making eye contact was some form of secret signal.

Then I got a grip on my pathetic fantasies, drank four large glasses of wine, and rolled home on the night bus to Mark.

The wave of lust doesn't only crash over me when it's someone new and shiny – it also hit me when I entered the flat and saw Mark sitting there playing Xbox in his pants. Hot and *accessible* – double whammy. I did my customary late-night collapse onto the carpet at his feet:

'Fun day?'

'Mmmfh.' I mumbled into a layer of shag-pile. The room was spinning slightly so I focused on him to try and balance myself – like when you stare at the horizon in a car to avoid feeling travel sick – staring at Mark helped to sober me up. He was almost totally immobile, save from his thick, sexy hands pressing buttons on the controller and the occasional shuffle to rearrange his dick.

'You're beautiful,' I muttered, and he nodded, smiling a simultaneous 'thanks' and 'you're a drunken eejit', and because he can grin both these messages at once, his smile is even better than the other guy's. Mark's shoulders, his arms, and everything else that's laid out so perfectly on the sofa gives me the same borderline-drooling lust that kicked me so heavily in the pub.

But it's not a comparison because it could never be. Just as Mark's wandering eye as he stands behind a girl on an escalator with a particularly lovely yoga-pants-clad bottom could never really be a comment on my own bottom. He'll get horny over other women in the same way as I do with men, yet somehow the idea of him actually acting on an impulse seems as odd to me as the idea that he'd sprout wings. When I was with Adam I tortured myself constantly with the idea of him finding someone else. I'd jealously hold him close to me when we were in female company, practically hissing like an alley cat if I sensed that spark of attraction. When Mark looks at other women, I feel good: 'She *is* pretty hot, so imagine what he thinks of me, the person he's chosen to be with!' He doesn't tell me other women are hot because he wants to hurt me, or because he's angling for some kind of threesome – he tells me because he trusts himself. He can say 'I saw this girl today with pink hair and dungarees' and know that there's no guilt in a crush if you never hope to act on it. It gives me an odd satisfaction, too – that he's let me into his fantasies so willingly I can easily pick out the kind of women who he'd consider 'his type'. Give me ten minutes and a pile of soft porn and I could happily sort it into pictures of people that Mark would either fuck or not fuck. And there'd be no jealousy, just a glow of pride. The confidence with which he can tell me who he fancies when we're sitting in a burlesque bar means I never find myself asking those small, painful questions – 'do you fancy her?' – the way I did with Adam. What's more, the fact that he can say 'Yeah, I'd shag Claire if she asked me to' means I'll never lie awake at night, wondering if he has. Indulging in this chat together is the closest I've ever come to understanding why I trust him. That night there was a vague idea in my spinning brain that I should tell him about the guy from earlier – open up like he does, and show I can share my own idle lusts as well.

While I was wondering whether to mention it, I fired up Twitter, scrolling idly through my timeline to find a girl he'd like: his type. Punky, small, with a 'fuck you' sneer. Or perhaps someone at the other end of the scale: calm, relaxed-looking, dressed in a T-shirt and no knickers, like she's tumbled out of bed on a hungover Saturday. It occurred to me that I could catalogue his different types in quite explicit detail, but only because he's been trusting enough to tell me when I've asked. I found a picture quite quickly, from a soft-porn Twitter feed that retweets cam girls who are looking for business. Wobbling a little, I held my phone up towards his face to show him the red-haired, small-breasted woman with the dark lips and the coy smile:

'Lovely,' he says. 'You're good at this.'

And the glow of pride feels so good that I don't tell him about earlier. I don't talk about the guy with the arm tattoo who made my cunt throb. There's nothing wrong with an idle crush, but I'm a coward and I don't want to spoil the moment.

I know it's not the end of the world if I look at a stranger with lust. Or even if I look at a stranger and temporarily forget that there's someone I know waiting at home in loose pyjamas, who'll give me the same feelings. Being in a relationship doesn't stop you fancying other people: that usually goes without saying. But I'm less likely to shout about what lies underneath: these feelings are powerful. After all, people *do* cheat. People break hearts and fuck strangers and have long, angsty conversations in the middle of the night about what their passion means – to shrug and say 'everyone has urges' is to downplay what the urges drive people to do. The more meaningless the crush seems, the harder it is to comprehend why someone would give in to it.

Fuck's sake – *I*. Why *I* gave in to it.

Seeing as I've started, let me reel off more of the same old excuses, because no guilt-ridden tryst is complete without them.

1. I was drunk. Obviously. Put a gigantic red tick in that box, then draw a tiny cocktail glass just to highlight that I wasn't normal-day drunk, I was unusually-cheap-cocktail-offers drunk. A heady mixture of new and interesting spinny sensations as well as new and interesting guys.
2. I was sad. This is always one, isn't it? Sad feelings are dramatic, so they make for a better excuse. It was one of those evenings I'd gone on to cheer myself up, and when you're on that kind of cheer-up mission, you're already neatly calibrated to ignore all alternative options in favour of grabbing the most selfish one.
3. Mark wasn't there.
4. I didn't actually have sex with anyone.

The squirmiest, measliest excuse of all, the one which hides all manner of sins. We've talked about what counts as cheating, but what technically 'counts' as sex anyway? Back at school there used to be heated discussion on whether it 'counted' if you lost your virginity but didn't come – while the boys nodded wisely, contemplating this seemingly philosophical question, we girls did our best to hold back gales of laughter. The question then moves on, when we're slightly older and more aware that there are people out there who aren't exactly the same as us, to the issue of gay sex. 'It can't just be about penetration, because lesbians lose their virginity too, right?' asks the smug bastard who thinks they're the first to have thought of it. 'And what about gay guys who don't like anal?' The answer, of course, is that there's no specific thing that 'counts' as losing one's virginity: for me it was having a penis in me for the first time (30 seconds to orgasm in a shed in his parents' garden. Obviously no orgasm for me: I am not a magic sex wizard), for others it might be oral, naked wriggling, or what have you. But the fact that sex is so broad and varied means that cheating fucks like me try to wriggle out on the specifics.

'Did you fuck him?' is, of course, an easy question to say 'Yes' or 'No' to. 'Did you cheat on me?' is harder, but as a general rule if you have to pause and think before replying, chances are your answer is 'Yes'.

Sorry – I'm stalling because I hate the next part.

It started with another guy who was my type and I think I'm closer to grasping just what puts him in that category. It wasn't in his smile or the casual way he knocked back whisky before leaning in to tell me a secret. It was what he said when he got there. A guy who tells me I'm beautiful or interesting wouldn't have the same effect. But a guy who tells me I'm a very dirty girl? Oh *god*.

Let's get this over with.

There are five of us, I think. Maybe six, maybe seven. It's late and I'm confused and we've been here a while. We went to see a show, on a Tuesday night. Tuesdays are safe, because normal people have work in the morning, so drinking themselves cross-eyed and getting home at 4am doesn't appeal, and regardless of what you might have heard about writers, I'm not going to do that on my own.

By 11pm the table is sticky – slicked with beer, cider, whisky, and sodden napkins with which we've halfheartedly attempted to clean up. The bell's already rung for last orders, and in our eagerness to continue a dark, vaguely sex-themed conversation, we miss our chance to get a final round in. When the barman comes over to gently usher us out of the bar, we exchange miserable looks. We're in our late 20s and early 30s – grown-ups with jobs and homes and responsibilities – yet the evening feels like a naughty treat, so we act accordingly: pouting and sulking like kids being called home for curfew.

'I know a cocktail bar near here,' someone says. 'I mean, I'm tired so I can probably only have one but...'

We're out of the door before she's even finished, staring into the distance like hounds who've scented blood. Except instead of blood it's sticky pink fizz that could be gin, vodka or Calpol: at this point none of us care. One couple peels away and heads for the tube station, then a few more depart, leaving just me, another girl and three guys I've only just met. Ignoring the buzzing in my pocket that means Mark is getting nervous, I decide I'll call him when we get there.

'There' turns out to be an inexplicably loud, hole-in-the-wall place, furnished with sticky sofas where we can sit close and smooshed together. I buy a round I can't afford and nudge myself in next to one particular person. Let's give him a name that's obviously not his real one: Michael. Michael is a looming nightmare, like the grey triangle you spot deep out to sea in a shark film before all hell breaks loose. Michael is tall, lithe, sarcastic, witty, clamouring for attention in a way that implies a need for sex. He has slim wrists and he wears a watch, and that combination of things fires the pervy part of my brain, giving me flash-frame visions of him wanking himself to completion: standing over me looking down at my tits, and jerking off until he comes. I can't even remember what we talked about, he could have been reciting his tax return for all I cared. I'm sure the chat turns sexual, though, because at one point he puts his hand on my neck and squeezes just the way I like it. Just because I asked him to.

Another guy – let's go with 'Owen', why not? – takes me outside for some fresh air. Where 'fresh air' naturally means 'chain-smoking cigarettes and chatting about bondage'. Turns out Owen is into submission: he likes women to tease and torment him, denying him pleasure and dishing out pain until he's bursting and squirming with forbidden joy. Of *course* I'm interested in Owen. He's nicer than Michael, who in turn is like me: doing the drunk thing where you're so keen to impress that you barely hear a word the other's saying. Sifting through their words to find an opportunity to buzz in. Owen makes jokes, asks questions and teases me for flirting, and if I didn't find his chat so hot I'd think I made a friend.

You don't need the gory details, do you? Or do you? At one point we got kicked out of the bar – possibly the first time in my life I'd actually heard someone utter the words 'Don't you lot have homes to go to?' – and we lost our other companions. The girl went home, the other bloke drifted off, and there we were: Owen, Michael, me, and a pathetically simple high consisting of booze and arousal, which none of us were ready to sleep off yet.

At the time it was delightful, I'm sure. The details which stuck with me in the taxi would all have worked for a wank: Michael's hands squeezing and pinching at me, Owen begging permission to bury his face into the soft suede of my boots. Me trying to gulp down half-hearted refusals then realising that Michael's hand around my throat felt too good for me to get the words out. A kiss, maybe. More likely a snatched semi-bite, his teeth gripping my bottom lip while Owen looked on. The moment I switched from passivity – a vague excuse to myself that none of this was my fault – to aggressive dominance. Giving Owen orders and holding out my boots for him to kiss. Pressing my lips against Michael's neck and pinching skin between my teeth. Dipping my fingers into my cunt and holding them out for them to lick.

As I say, it was hot at the time. And it's my job now to make it sound hotter still – to play up the clit-throbbing, urgent *lust* of it. But no matter how delicious the details, it will always sound sordid, because it was. The sober truth is miserable and small: three horny drunks gathered somewhere in North London – no hotel rooms or bondage bars or fetish parties – just a bench by the roadside, a few honking taxi drivers, and a quick and dirty fumble up against a tree. One guy choking me while the other licked at my boots. All the while my phone's buzzing guilt in my pocket and I'm stacking up misery for Mark to swallow later, when I limp home at dawn with the start of a hangover and a trembling, wretched confession.

It's not even a worthwhile crime: not a threesome with hot strangers or a holiday fuck I'll remember forever, just a giggling mistake. It's certainly not worth Mark's forgiveness, which he duly gives me the next day, holding me like it was an accident that happened *to* me rather than a mistake I made on my own.

For the next two weeks I make the coffee again, and I feel exactly as shit as I deserve to. Love might mean being forgiven your mistakes, but somehow the forgiveness feels finite. After all, if this didn't hurt Mark then it wouldn't need to be forgiven. If we were in an open relationship, then the only crime would have been not answering my phone, but as it is there's something much bigger and darker to contend with. When Mark strokes my hair, shaking to hold back his own tears, he tells me that this one's bigger than last time. Not because he needs me to hurt, but because he needs me to know that *he* does. He hurts because I didn't say no. He hurts because he was worried and scared and wanted to know I was safe. But above all because he's realised that repeatedly forgiving each small betrayal has made me more selfish, not less. It hurts him because this time he really *does* know what I'm thinking: not 'I shouldn't have done it' but 'I should have made it worth it'. I spent some of Mark's forgiveness on... this?

What a waste.

How To Decide Whether Or Not To Have A Baby: 13 Steps

(wikihow.com)

Him: Shall we get married?
Me: Why?
Him: Payback for all the people who make us go to ***their*** *weddings.*

If this really were a rom-com, one of two things would happen: either Mark and I would split up, or we'd have a dramatic reunion in which we declared our undying love for each other. If you're my mum, you're probably rooting for the latter. If you're after the former, perhaps you're holding out for someone other than Mark to come along, making way for an ending crammed with juicy sex scenes, in which I fuck my way through London zones 2 and 3, before coming to rest in a jizz-slathered heap somewhere on a Central Line tube at dawn.

We're actually going somewhere a bit different: a cheap Mexican restaurant, in which Mark and I are sipping weird-flavoured margaritas and having a lovely chat about The Future.

I like talking about The Future. It's one of the very few conversations I can have with Mark and no one else. If other people ask 'Are you going to get married?' it feels intrusive, like someone's popped up in your living room and asked what colour your pants are. If Mark asks me it feels collaborative – more like a strategy meeting for two eager yet incompetent professionals. Sometimes The Future involves discussions like the ones we had after the drunken fumbling incident – long nights of soul searching that have no tangible conclusion. While I'd love the drama of a big fight or cathartic make-up sex, in reality neither of these things happened. The days drifted on, and we kept loving each other and without making a conscious choice about it, we sealed that problem in a box and hid it away, hoping it would disappear if we left it for long enough. I know that's not always the right move, but it's part of the weird dichotomy of being a grown up: you want to be adult about things, and you feel you know the right way to do it, but a teeny bit of you would rather just eat ice cream for breakfast and pretend that the scary bits aren't happening. The discussion about cheating will come out again eventually, but for now we've decided that there's something more interesting to explore: we're having fun playing at grown-ups. What if, instead of wondering when we'll split up, we consider what happens if we *don't?*

Mark's theory of relationships, rather than being a mishmash of lust, confusion and swear words, is pretty damn simple:

we are two separate units playing on the same team. Mark has his personal goals (get a job where he can buy Haribos on expenses) and I have mine (make my blog graphs go up and avoid being 'discovered' by a guy with a throat-bleeding fetish), we also have a few of those coveted shared goals that we can fight for together.

Over burritos and margaritas, Team Sarah and Mark are assessing roughly where they're up to. They've managed to move in together (tick!), get a joint mortgage (tick!) and avoid burning the house down (given his forgetfulness and my paranoia, we see this as a significant victory). Mark is the first to raise the question of what happens next, and judging by his reaction, he thinks my own list is desperately mundane. Mine consists of:

1. Go on holiday. We haven't been on holiday since a long weekend to Kiev three years ago, during which we had sex in a see-through bath tub and we failed to go to Chernobyl.
2. Build a shed in the garden, so that I become a real writer.
3. Buy a sofa that we can have sex on without it making creaking noises.

He humours me, with a yes to one and three and a maybe on the writing shed:

'Our neighbours will see inside, so you'll have to stop taking midday wank breaks in case they call the council.'

'We could get blinds?' I suggest, and he shakes his head.

'Why would someone close the blinds in their office in the middle of the day unless they were wanking? You might as well call it "Shuffler's Cottage" and have done with it.'

'OK. So no shed. What do *you* think we should do next?'

His ambitions are a little bigger. Or rather they're smaller, fleshier and come with a startling array of accessories.

'Not right now,' he begins, sensibly. 'But one day. Babies?'

'Argh.' It's not a 'no' – not a flat-out 'no', and for that I'm quite proud of myself. In my head I give me a 'well done for being brave' badge. 'Hmm. What answer are you looking for here?'

'Well, judging by previous times we've had this conversation,' he begins, 'I think you say "we'll see", followed by a long diatribe on how the idea of being pregnant terrifies you, topped off with a quick round of "why am I only considered to have succeeded as a woman if I push a small infant out of my body?" Then we get drunk and forget about it for another six months.'

'You know me so well.'

But this time I'm up for it. Not the babies – the conversation. We've had variations on it before, but never ones that have given me cause to run for the hills, because I fend them off before they get serious. About nine months after we started dating we had a long, stoned debate about the merits of having children. Mark explained why he wants them and I got rabidly defensive. It's easy enough for a guy to say he's always wanted children, because he can have them as an 'and' alongside his other wants. As a general rule, I get to pick them as an option in an either/or battle: my freedom and career on one side, tiny baby bootees on the other. If, like Mark, I could have kids without pregnancy, keep my job, and get a pat on the back for doing the odd feed or walk in the park, I'd jump at the chance to have them too.

I know Mark better now than I did then, though. He'd never be the kind of dad who passed a kid over as soon as it wet its nappy. We're more ready for The Future chat now, it's easier to imagine what kind of small creature the two of us would create. Nerdy, of course, but outspoken in the right context. My strong opinions but with Mark's calm voice. And surely, with enough encouragement (I'd be a fun mum! I'm sure I would!), any kid we brought up would get a love of maths from Mark and a love of words from me. Maybe it would even get a combination of our looks that wouldn't cause it to have a permanently startled expression – we're in doubt about that though.

'It *might* be cute.' I try to ease into the 'fuck no' that both of us know is coming, by conceding on this minor point.

'Of course it would be cute: it'd have me for a dad. And if it wasn't cute then I'd teach it to be cute by batting its eyelashes and charming its mummy until she agreed to do things she'd never have thought of doing before.'

'Who'd look after it, though?'

'Both of us.'

Good idea in theory: Team Mark and Sarah can do quite a bit when we put our heads together, and perhaps looking after a baby is one of those things. But in practice Mark taking on half of the childcare is nothing *like* an easy option. We live in a world where, in the average office, he would earn about 15% more than me for doing the same job. Where men looking after their children are frequently referred to as 'babysitting'. Where, despite his occasional Herculean efforts to pick up a dishcloth, I still end up doing the majority of the housework. Not because, as Mark claims, he just doesn't 'see' that there's washing up which needs to be done, but because over the course of 30-odd years he's been repeatedly told that it's not his job to do it. In case he starts sounding like an unreconstructed bastard, and I like a nagging shrew, I should point out that we're both aware of this, and work hard to address it. Our home life doesn't consist of Mark scratching his balls while I hoover under his feet, occasionally shrieking 'patriarchy!' when he forgets to move them. OK, maybe that does happen *sometimes*. But so do days where Mark falls into a whirlpool of guilt and spends hours scrubbing the oven clean because he wants to contribute his share but can't quite work out what needs to be done. And the odd day where I just shout 'fuck it!' and hurl all his dirty clothes into a passive-aggressive pile at the end of the bed, wishing there were enough socks to spell out 'do the laundry you shitbag' on the floor.

We started with children and we've wandered into dirty socks territory, but for a really good reason: children and dirty socks are inextricably linked together. Not just because kids produce a hell of a lot of laundry, but because the very act of looking after children is, like housework, usually considered 'women's work'. It would be phenomenally sexist of me to let Mark off the hook when it comes time to share the chores: saying 'oh baby, you're such a *man*' if he forgets to do any of the tedious, menial tasks that prevent our house from turning into a plague pit. When all the household chores are added together, I spend roughly ten hours a week cooking, cleaning, tidying, sorting, and screaming silent screams into my pillow because holy Christ this is not what I want to do with my life. Then, when I have finished with the screaming and I get into a bit of a moan, people tell me that it isn't important: 'Oh, it's *only* the washing up,' they say, as if I'm arguing that it's actually rocket science. It's not, of course, but as a general rule rocket scientists become rocket scientists because they *want* to: they've chosen a path, and they get the respect that comes from being able to construct a rocket that'll fly to the moon. No one ever sat me down and said 'Hey, do you fancy doing the majority of unpaid labour in your household from adolescence until the day you croak, with barely any thanks and absolutely no option to ever stop?'

With children, on the other hand, I *do* have a choice. They don't just get dropped off by the stork, babies are like vampires: you have to invite them in. Just as I can choose to get a dishwasher and thus do slightly less washing up, so I can choose not to have children and thus never be put in the position where I'm changing nappies ten times a day and begging Mark to do 'just one or two – to show you're trying'.

'I *would* look after them, you know.' Mark's hurt, and understandably. When I get on my high horse he often gets trampled, and I should learn to pull back a bit. He didn't personally create this mess and he has to deal with the fallout from it too. One of the reasons this conversation is so difficult for both of us is that we were both told it would happen the other way round: I should be panting in baby-related anticipation, and Mark should be charmingly nervous of kids, Hugh Granting his way through excuses and 'dear oh dear I don't think I'm readys'. As you can probably guess, what with his excessive desire for cuddles and his desire to maintain an actual relationship as opposed to a housemates-who-shag scenario, Mark's pretty keen on commitment. If you mention the c-word he's less likely to run for the hills than to rummage through the Ikea catalogue, excitedly planning what the nursery will look like. Instead of dreading it as any normal human (i.e. me) would, he actively looks forward to those classes where they teach pregnant women how to breathe, showing toddlers to use their legs and loudly shushing relatives when they accidentally swear at a wedding. My future dreams are all about dirty weekends, wanking sheds and sofas we can fuck on without creaking, and it feels inappropriate to usher children into that. Yet regardless of our individual desires, I'm treated like 'Cruella DeVille' when I say I don't want children, and Mark's treated with caution when he says he's looking forward to them.

When we visit friends who've had babies, the same thing always happens:

'Would you like a cuddle?' they ask me – *just* me – in the syrupy voice we all use around children, because children have secret powers that cause us all to gurgle like they do.

'Sure,' I say, reaching out and grabbing armfuls of sticky infant. I feel proud for about ten seconds that I've managed to hold one without dropping it and that it made a face at me which could plausibly be interpreted as a smile. Then it starts crying and I look around in panic. If Mark's next to me I'll hand it to him, so he can perform whichever of his everyday miracles causes babies to go calm in his arms. At this point the parent usually looks confused – why would *Mark* want to hold the baby? Occasionally, heartbreakingly, they look suspicious – men don't know what they're doing! Don't trust an incompetent *man* with my precious bundle of joy!

When we're in company, Mark will explain his love of kids with the easy, macho excuses that people expect:

'If I'm holding a baby, I don't have to talk to any grown-ups.' Then grown-ups nod and feel a bit sorry for the shy guy who's uncomfortable making small talk. But alone with me he'll give a bit more detail: babies are cute. They have teeny hands. It's nice to hang out with a human who only cares about whether they're comfy and there's milk to hand. He conjures a picture of a baby which is half him and half me, and I have to admit it's cute to imagine it falling asleep on his chest. If we had a child of our own, he could teach it all the things that he teaches me. How to chill out. How to play Xbox. How to calculate the bill split in restaurants. How to draw on a seemingly endless well of patience. How to love without nit-picking about the details. If he was the baby's father, he wouldn't have his child snatched away after five minutes, to be handed instead to a woman. If you think that we've made strides in terms of gender equality and childcare, then please join me in celebrating the things we *have* done that are valuable: in the UK parents now have better options for shared parental leave, which mean childcare can be more evenly split no matter what the genders of the couple. We've started to ditch the excesses of gender-split clothes, where girl babies are clad exclusively in saccharine pink and boys given trucks and blue things. But we're still far from perfect: just watch what happens next time you're in a mixed-gender group and someone's passing round a baby.

When we've had a good old bitch about this, over our third margarita and a dessert of cinnamon churros, Mark picks up the previous thread and skilfully nudges me towards more concrete answers. Should we? Will we? When?

'I'm not saying you *have* to have kids, I am saying that I still think I want to.'

'I know. You're good with kids.'

'Damn right I'm good with kids.'

'They're your intellectual equals, after all.'

'Stop pissing about.' Fair point. 'Look: I know all the arguments against it – you hate the idea of being pregnant and having one of those whatsits...'

'Episiotomy.'

'Right. Epelioctomy. Whatever.'

'Not "whatever", Mark – they cut your fanny with scissors!'

'I know. And that's shit. But I'm trying to list things here to show I'm listening. So: pregnancy is bad. Children mean more housework. You don't like the idea that you have to have kids to be a success as a woman. And... what was the other one?'

'Kids are expensive and time-consuming. I'd prefer to go on holiday.'

'Right.' There's a *but* coming. I can sense it. Everything about Mark's body language says *but...* – from the way he folds his napkin and places it on the table, to the serious, pleading eyes he turns on me.

'But,' I *knew* it. 'Thing is, I still think I want children.'

Yeah, that's a kicker. Mark's not trying to put pressure on me. He's definitely not telling me what so many other parents do: 'You'll change your mind one day' or, worse: 'Have them while you can because you'll regret it if you don't.' Bizarre conversations like that tend to ramp up after your 30th birthday and I can't help but be baffled and ever-so-slightly horrified by them (a friend once told me, during her second round of IVF, that I should try for kids now anyway because 'one day it will be too late', and I was torn between sympathy and terror. I should have kids now, *even though I don't want any*, in case I decide I like them in the future? That's not a decision you make about a baby, that's a decision you make about a pair of boots that you spotted in the sale). She means well, of course, but I'm not sure how many of the people who tell me I'll 'change my mind' understand just how often I've heard this. Others don't realise how aggressive they sound when they regurgitate one of the more extreme arguments: it's 'selfish' not to have children, or it's your 'only purpose on this planet' to reproduce. It's neither of these things, of course, there are plenty of ways to contribute to the world other than by putting new people in it, and it would only be 'selfish' not to have them if kids were in limited supply. So why are people so desperate to persuade strangers that they have to give birth? Laying aside for a moment the huge gulf between what men are told ('Don't blame you mate, lot of hassle!') and what women are told ('But motherhood is practically sacred!') my theory is that it's all about justifying your own choices. For a long time we (and women in particular) have been led to believe that there's no real choice in the matter: through biological imperative, cultural conditioning, or just because they're so damn cute, everyone was taught that babies should come as standard. Now that it's becoming clearer there's a choice, someone choosing not to have them isn't seen for what it is – just one different option among many. It's often interpreted as a personal insult. As with relationships, those who are monogamous are usually keen to extol the benefits of their own system and tell others why it's the 'best' way. Likewise with children, some people who have picked option 'A' see me choosing 'B' and leap to the dreadful possibility that I think their choice is wrong. Why do they do this? Because for so long it's only ever been presented as a 'right/wrong' choice. My parents, for example, would have been told they were wrong if they chose not to have kids. My grandparents too and so on back through the generations to my great-great grandmother, who no doubt hardly thought about it. Because of this, introducing new options looks, to people who are happily enjoying the status quo, like their choice is being taken away. It's not being taken away though, parents, I promise: it's just that not everyone's picking it. It certainly feels more secure when everyone's in your camp, but in the long run it's better if we spread out a bit – take different paths and accept that what's right for you might be wrong for me, and vice versa. There's no answer sheet that we all have to get right. Besides, if I don't have kids I'll have way more money to spend on nephews and nieces at Christmas. I'm a really fun auntie when I'm sober.

This is perhaps why Mark's the only one I can talk to seriously about children. Until it's generally accepted that being childless can be a legitimate choice, that conversation will always be bogged down in politics. With Mark, though, we can strip away all the politics and expectations and focus purely on what each of us wants. Mark wants to have children. I don't.

'Tell you what,' he says, because he's always better at putting a full-stop to things than I am, 'I'll just ask once every six months or so – check in on how you're feeling about it. You never know, one of us might change our mind.'

It's the 'one of us' that gets me. There's a nagging feeling that no matter how long I put it off, soon it'll be time to make a choice – if I genuinely love Mark, and want to be a Real Grown-Up, then perhaps I'll have to accept some of the grown-up, mature stuff that I've been putting off until now.

The other option is unthinkably sad: if Mark and I want radically different futures, then what's the point in us having a present?

When we get home, we fuck the way we always do and yet I can't help but think of conception. There's nothing gentle or soft or purposeful about it: I grind against him until I'm raw, gritting my teeth and squeezing my eyes tight – trying to focus on the sensations, but it all feels forced. I'd only just got my head around the idea that sex was an expression of love, now I'm being asked to go one further and imagine sperm meeting egg, and toddlers marching headlong into the bedroom and ruining all my fun.

When Lucy told me the story of how she and her husband conceived (not with positions and diagrams, although that would have made for a brilliant baby shower), I'd found it hard to comprehend the idea of getting pregnant *deliberately*. My entire life has been one long quest to find the perfect contraception: condoms, tablets, coils, and the occasional panicked trip to the chemists to buy a morning after pill and a cider to wash it down with. Since I was 15, the message was always 'don't get pregnant!' complete with bright neon exclamation mark and wagging finger. It was 'don't muck up your life' and 'you're not old enough for children' and 'kids ruin everything!' I can't pinpoint the exact moment when it flipped from those doom-laden warnings to the urgent instruction to 'have babies now!' but there was one. There's no middle-ground phase to give you time to consider the options, just a dire warning that gives way to an urgent deadline. Instructions to steer clear of the edge are replaced with orders to jump straight off it.

15 Romantic Gestures For Him To Feel Your Love

(*youqueen.com*)

Him: We're not boring, we've just realised it's more fun to stay at home and swear at each other than go out and swear in the pub.

Don't look now – we're nearly at the end of the book and Mark and I are still together! I know it's a shaky, uncertain, will-they-won't-they kind of together. But we're together nonetheless.

If you're with someone I'm sure you'll understand. The idea of 'forever' is simultaneously exciting and appalling, and the feeling of it can change from one minute to the next. Good times feel perfect: a sign! This will definitely last forever! Then something minor happens and you plunge into a bad time: a sign! We're going to split up and we haven't paid off the new bathroom yet! Neither of these things has to be massive, either. In films and stories the highs are always really high (a proposal! A baby!) and the lows are appalling (a break-up! One of them killed the other one's dog!), but in reality the good signs can be as simple as a giggling fit at a summer festival or a nice gesture on a rainy day. Mark and I are big fans of festivals, mainly because we enjoy sweaty tent sex, and eating jacket potatoes at four in the morning. One Saturday summer evening, we lounged on the grass in a festival arena, listening to a band I'd never heard of and soaking up the joy of being drunk and happy. Two days with no phone reception had left me remarkably calm, and I'd slowed my pace to match his. But out of the corner of his eye he spotted something that made him sit up sharply and nudge me. Uncharacteristically wound up, he hissed: 'Do you see that? It's an outrage!' He pointed to a woman sitting on a blanket nearby: 40-ish, two young children and a couple of friends. In her lap she had a huge basket, out of which she pulled a selection of delicious picnic-y treats: cheese, bread, that kind of thing. Mark's face was a picture of faux-outrage.

'She's got... *wine*!'

'So?'

'In *glass bottles*. In the *main arena*.'

His exaggerated anger was simultaneously hilarious, adorable and utterly righteous. As he explained, in whispers so her children didn't hear, it simply wasn't fair: there were kids outside the arena being made to throw away cans of Strongbow because you couldn't bring in alcohol. Yet this woman – 'this fooking *twat*' – had managed to sneak past security with a hamper filled with wine. Never normally one to play by the rules, Mark was suddenly livid at the entitlement of a neat and organised lady having a picnic at a festival. Something about his sunburned face, twisted into a look of utter disgust at this middle-class injustice, set me off into fits of giggles.

'It's not just one, she's got two *different* wines! A selection of wines! I have never been so angry in my life.' I buried his head in my stomach to muffle my laughter, as he kept up a stream of expletives in his lilting northern accent. Just as I calmed down, he started again: 'I don't believe it – she's got fucking *chutney*!'

Moments like that, when Mark is at his sarcastic, adorable best, can be so wonderful that the idea of staying with him makes me Christmas-morning excited. If you'd asked me in that moment how I felt about Mark I'd have given you platitudes: he's funny, brilliant, the love of my life. Likewise if you asked me on another good day – the Sunday he walked into the living room to find me watching *Rain Man*. I'd been struggling for a few weeks – too much work and not enough sleep and that ever-present buzz of panic. While he had a lie-in I decided to take a rare couple of hours away from writing to lie on the sofa and relax. It hurt a bit, and I'm not good at relaxing. Sometimes I need him to hold me tightly just to help me stop fidgeting. But this time I'd done it voluntarily, and I was pretty bloody pleased with myself. My brain still told me to get on with work, but my body was on strike: I sat beneath a blanket, arranged my limbs the way I thought a calm person would, and watched the film. Mark woke up about halfway through the film, and sauntered through into the living room in his dressing gown.

'Morn... wait. Are you *relaxing*?'

'Yep.'

'Like I told you to?'

'Yep.'

He grinned, then hurried out. Twenty minutes later he came back with a pile of grapes, a bag of chocolate buttons and four cans of cheap cider. He unloaded the gifts on the table, whispered 'you're such a good girl' and then tiptoed out of the room.

There are so many days like these: not significant like a birthday or a holiday, just quietly exceptional moments when you think your other half's perfect. It's what you expect once you've walked into the sunset: calm, idyllic moments of support. But equally there are days that make 'the rest of our lives' sound ominous. If you asked me what I thought of Mark after a long day sitting on the sofa, watching crap sci-fi when I was desperate to go outside, I'd have been less keen. If you asked him when we were on our way out, me tapping my foot and snarling as he delayed us by another hour, he'd probably have said the same. During that one big row where he retreated to the bath to drink whisky and I stormed off to my mum's house with a bag full of clothes and a head full of confusion, we'd probably both have guessed it was The End.

Depending on the day, the idea of our entire lives stretching before us as one long Saturday-afternoon-on-the-sofa can either feel like heaven or jail. On paper-scissors-stone day? Heaven again. When I'm hoovering? Jail. The problem with humans is that they come in a mixture of awful as well as awesome. The rom-com can never really capture this, because in order to suck you in it has to persuade you that the heroes are perfect. When the leading man sings a love song to the leading lady, he will gamely forget the row they had the other night because she threw out his favourite jacket. Her face won't show how bitter she is that he wore that ratty old thing during Christmas dinner with her parents. It wouldn't be as heart warming if we knew how much he interrupted her, or how irritating she could be when she didn't get her own way.

I have never sung a love song to Mark, or even performed an impromptu comedy set just for him at a festival. Nor have I taken him for a dirty weekend, or persuaded a bunch of friends to learn a complicated dance routine so I can propose to him and get a million hits on YouTube. While he'd love me to take on any traditional romantic gesture, I don't think I've even given him flowers. If we're in this 'forever' zone – the one that's supposed to feel like happy ever after – then shouldn't I do something to show him that I'm glad to be here? Unfortunately, while I'm more mature than I was on that Wednesday, when the combination of anxiety and doubt meant that what should have been nice felt like prison, I still suck at romance. When Mark's birthday rolls around again I stare blankly at a bunch of Lego toys on Amazon wondering if I can get away with just closing my eyes and hitting the 'buy now' button on anything vague and playful. I still end up declaring my romantic intentions via drunk text messages or scribbled limericks about his cock.

It's not like I'm totally incapable, though. I have hazy memories of romantic acts I committed in the past, to varying degrees of success. I once made a mix tape for a boy I adored, handing it to him with a flourish and praying inside that he'd be so touched by the songs that I'd chosen, he'd strip naked and leap dick-first into my bed. I spent weeks afterwards expecting him to make reference to the tape. I dropped hints about it to solicit comments, and played the right CDs at parties to see if he'd say 'oh, I remember this from the mix tape, it's one of my favourites, please allow me to hump you passionately in the airing cupboard', or at the very least come and snog me while we danced. But he did neither of these things: he simply *never mentioned it*.

I haven't had much luck with flowers either. I once bought a guy a blue rose, and I can tell you're impressed already – the playful nature of a single rose, combined with the surprise that it's blue – I mean, who ever heard of a blue rose? Unfortunately, if you scratch beneath the surface you'll see that this wasn't an 'I love you' so much as a 'Fuck you'. This particular guy and I had been arguing about whether or not blue roses existed. So, when I spent ages hunting down a blue one and triumphantly presenting it to him, I felt like I was not only showing effort but also ticking those 'shared in-joke' boxes that make romantic gestures more special. Unfortunately, as I handed it to him, I forgot that the whole point was to be cute, and I ended up crowing 'See? They DO exist! I was RIGHT!' A week later, as the water in the vase started to turn blue as well, I got the sneaking suspicion I'd been ripped off.

I'd love to do a similar thing for Mark, only without the smugness and with a far better rose. Problem is, he's already done the 'rose' thing, and he managed to pull it off with far more placid dignity than I could. He came home from work, shouted 'Where are you?' then dumped a bouquet of yellow roses on the kitchen counter.

'Ooh, blimey, thanks! These are nice.'

'Yeah. Nicer than your face.'

Then we hugged, fucked, cooked dinner and put the telly on.

I have done one or two grand gestures too, by which I mean 'expensive'. I booked a romantic holiday for Adam once. Long weekend, so you're probably thinking Paris. But we were young and horny and I was too tight for Paris. Besides, my French barely stretches further than 'pain au chocolat', so we'd probably have come home with diabetes. Thus: Amsterdam. Long days of museum hopping, dodging trams and being screamed at by angry cyclists, followed by evenings in which we'd get enthusiastically stoned and fuck quickly in those porno DVD booths. The two of us crowded into a small wooden cubicle that smelled strongly of other people's spunk, he'd sit on the sticky wooden bench and I'd sit on his lap with my skirt lifted and knickers pushed to one side. I'd ride his cock while he fed Euros into the slot to keep the porn playing. When I came, he'd put his hand over my mouth to stop me from crying out, and when *he* came I'd drop to my knees and swallow it, to save us leaving the place even grimier than it was when we entered. Then we'd head back to a dark coffee shop until we were horny enough to go again. It was one of my favourite holidays, although I probably wouldn't explain *exactly* why in a TripAdvisor review.

Sadly, while the holiday itself ticked the perfect 'staged-kidnap-style' romance boxes, it failed to do much for him. I'd hoped that when I revealed the surprise, he'd react with delight. After all, I'd forked out a bunch of money, spent meticulous hours planning, and even worked out a great way to reveal the surprise to him – I was expecting to get my money's worth in squeals of pleasure and declarations of undying love. Unfortunately, he must have been in a bit of a shit mood, because when I told him about the trip – producing an Amsterdam guidebook with a flourish, and anticipating immediate gratitude sex – all he said was:

'I've never thought about going to Amsterdam,' followed by a long and painful silence.

I swallowed down the lump that was growing in my throat, threatening to make me look like a miserable prick and explained, 'I thought this might be a cool thing for us to do together.'

'You probably can't afford it,' he said, handing the guide book back to me.

'I can! I've paid for it already!'

'Oh, really? OK, we'll have to go then.'

Ouch.

At the time I was utterly crushed – my amazing gesture! My wonderful plan! And he couldn't even *pretend* to be pleased? If he sounds like an arse, I promise he wasn't. I wanted a reward just for making the effort, which is the equivalent of buying flowers from a petrol station then getting angry that I hadn't earned a shag. It was very early days in our relationship, and while *I* felt like a weekend away was exactly the right investment (and I'd have spent double my student loan for just *one* good fuck in a porn booth), he saw the extravagance as a worrying sign of disparity in our affections. I hadn't just given him tickets, but the obligation to use and enjoy them with me, when he may have preferred to stay home.

The success of any given romantic gesture often comes down to how well it's received. A friend of mine once told me a story about a guy she knew, who was madly in love with one of his friends. He journeyed the two hours it took him by train to turn up at her house, then rather than knocking on the door and sobbing his undying love directly, he decided to be a bit more subtle. He knew she was a chess lover, so he left two chess pieces – a king and a queen – on her doorstep, along with a dozen red roses and a note explaining how he felt.

'Aww,' I said. 'That's romantic.'

'Fuck that,' she replied. 'It is creepy as hell.'

The thing is, told a different way, that reads like the story of a man who is so obsessed with a girl that he takes a long and arduous journey to the place where she lives: strike one in the 'stalker' list. He then declares his undying love for her by leaving her a note on the doorstep, thus not only saying 'I know where you live' in the manner of a serial killer, but also making her feel like she has to respond in some way. Strike three – he's making reference to something she loves so that he can say 'See? I *know* you...' with the chilling implication 'Because I've been watching...' It's the old 'charming stalker' conundrum: that the language of love is eerily similar to the language of dangerous obsessives – why else would Sting's 'I'll be Watching You' get played so frequently at wedding discos? You could read almost any monologue from a romantic novel or play and hear it at both ends of the spectrum. Spoken aloud down the phone with a voice distorter, even 'Shall I compare thee to a summer's day?' sounds like reason to call the police.

In real life, the difference between being a stalker and being romantic is fairly easy to spot – like the difference between sex and rape, it's all down to mutual consent. We don't initiate sex by turning up naked on the doorstep of someone we fancy and start eagerly tonguing them: we chat, and ask and whisper dirty stories, and only step things up a gear when we're pretty sure they're up for it. Likewise with romance – you don't spot a hot guy on the bus and immediately surprise him with Eurostar tickets to Paris, you start with the little things. My first boyfriend got smudged letters declaring my undying devotion ('What does that say? I can't read your writing'), other boyfriends have received small tokens that I've picked up in shops because 'I saw this and thought of you' (or, more honestly, 'I saw this and thought of your penis').

While Adam was grumpy about our Amsterdam trip, he responded much better to smaller gestures: a couple of pretty excellent poems and a hand-drawn cartoon card. Ignoring the fact that I draw about as well as a dog licking an inkwell, the cartoon card was a stroke of genius because it illustrated one of our many fights and came with a message that essentially read 'I hope you don't mind that I'm a bit of a nob'. Once or twice I even got him tickets to his favourite bands, despite the fact that I'd rather lie face-down on a pavement all night than stand up for two hours at a gig. The gesture was there to say 'I love you so much I'll do this thing I hate': I'd do it and hate it and smile all the way through, then get fucked at the end to reward me for my patience. Yet with Mark I've done little more than buy him chocolate and packets of love hearts. If I want to say 'I love you' with anything other than words, there has to be something he actually *wants*.

Is there anything?

'Yes.'

'Oooh, what?'

'Pizza.'

'Pizza?'

'Yes. Let's order in pizza.'

'No, I mean bigger than that. Like the kind of thing I'd get you for your birthday.'

'Pizza.' He grins. This is not a wind-up grin, this is a grin that is genuinely excited for pizza, and cannot comprehend that there could be something better.

'OK, we'll get pizza. But anything else? I mean something special, that only I can give y —'

'Blow job.' That grin again. Pizza and a blow job. Eyebrows raised ever so slightly as if to say 'maybe I could have both at the same time?'

'We... umm... can do that. I was thinking something *even better* as well though.'

'You want something that's better than pizza and a blow job *at the same time*? Good luck with that!' He kisses me, and chuckles, and goes back to watching TV.

We're back with the birthday conundrum: Mark just loves the way life is now. Not only are all his basic needs met, but his whims are fulfilled with an alarming efficiency. At three in the afternoon he'll email me a link to a cool set of magnets on Amazon. 'We can use these to fix the kitchen cupboard!' he exclaims excitedly. The next morning, while I'm putting in an order for the magnets his heart desires, the doorbell will go and they'll arrive, along with a weeding tool for the garden, 12 portable battery packs, a box of sweets and a cowboy hat. This is the week before his next birthday, and because magnets are crossed off the wish list, I field desperate emails from members of his family, who have no idea what to buy him – what do you get the man who won't wait 24 hours for a set of magnets and a cowboy hat? I dispense vague guesses based on his recent whims and on the day there's a flurry of deliveries containing, in ascending order of weirdness: a laptop stand, a build-it-yourself robotic hand, and an actual, honest-to-god axe. Mark is equally delighted with all of them, and sets about chopping up bits of the garden while laughing like a supervillain.

'How about tickets to a show?'

'That's what *you* like.'

'A camping trip?'

'Ditto.'

'OK, but what do *you* like? If you had a day and could go anywhere...?'

'Here,' he says, pointing to the sofa, then pulling me face-first into his comfortable crotch.

So there you have it: I've never done anything good for Mark. Not a dirty weekend (he'd prefer the sofa), or a half-burned breakfast in bed (he'd rather sleep till two). I could just give him a blow job while he eats a pizza and have done with it, but I want to do something significant. After all the miracles he's worked for me, I'd quite like to present him with a gesture that, if not YouTube-worthy, at least gives him something to remember in a year's time when yet again we're fighting over what to watch on Netflix. Something he can cling to in the shit moments, that'll carry him through my fuck-ups, in the same way as I float through his by remembering roses and *Rain Man*.

How to Be A Rebel: 13 Steps

(With Pictures) (*wikihow.com*)

Me: If you were a time traveller, would you go back in time and have sex with yourself?
Him: Dunno. I think I could do better, to be honest.

When I was younger I used to wear a lot of make-up. I say 'make-up' but what I actually mean is 'face paint' – the traditional pasty-white goth face with eyeliner used as substitute lipstick. Within an hour of leaving the house (in black corduroy trousers, a black T-shirt and homemade belt-chain from this season's B&Q collection), everything would start flaking off. By 5 o'clock, what hadn't been smeared on a collar or mashed onto my teenage boyfriend's face would clump together and make me look like I had a skin condition. Nevertheless, I was delighted with it. Not because I thought I looked good (although now I positively *ache* to be that person again, because life is cruel and we all want what's already gone), I just knew I looked dramatic enough that the guys I liked would pause for a second look. They'd usually decide, in that look, that I was a bit too weird or my teeth were slightly dodgy, but at least I'd have had a moment of heart-soaring joy knowing that they'd looked in the first place.

If you'd asked me whether I cared about make-up I'd have told you I didn't.

'I hate make-up,' I'd have explained, and then added like a judgemental twat: 'It's just a way for women to make themselves all look the same.' Add whatever other bullshit arguments you can here – if you're stuck you'll find millions of them posted online beneath young girls' instagram selfies. 'It's shallow.' 'It's pointless.' 'It's expensive.' 'It's a reflection of how you're not interesting enough as a person that you have to rely on your looks.' All that bollocks. Yet I still wore it – a deliberate pastiche of the more popular stuff that my peers would shoplift from Boots, but make-up nonetheless. The irony of this non-rebellion, while lost on my teenage self, doesn't escape me now: it's all very well to kick back against what's expected, but if I pretend that doing the exact *opposite* means I'm some kind of superstar, I am hopelessly wrong.

Like goth-Sarah slapping on terrifying make-up, grown-up Sarah smashes out terrifying blog posts and articles decrying the way the world tries to put us neatly into little boxes. Like goth-Sarah, she's probably right that we shouldn't all feel we have to dress/look/fuck/live the same, but she has crappy ideas about what we should do instead. Just as no one wants a world full of Stepford wives, in neatly pressed aprons and flawless natural make-up, so no one wants to live in a world of teenage goths either. Imagine the miserable music! The lack of colour! The soaring cost of fishnet tights!

Our relationship myths matter because for every happy Stepford wife there'll be a lonely goth wondering why she's been forced into this pinafore, wanting to douse her Cath Kidston tea towel in kerosene and burn the world to the ground. But that doesn't make the smug goth inherently *better* than the person who's happily baking, or the millions of others who fall somewhere in between on this weird goth/Stepford spectrum. Not only is there a genuine spectrum, for almost any choice I can think of, but people can move up and down it whenever they like. Claire can one minute be the happily married woman, and the next be shuffling Tinder dates and wondering how best to celebrate her divorce. Lucy is having babies now, happily ensconced with her husband in a world where everything's homemade and smells like fresh baking. I can moan about commitment and struggle to come up with a gesture more romantic than that blow job/pizza combo, but that doesn't mean that any one of us should be a template for the other.

A lot of the questions we ask about sex and love come down to this obsession with binary things. Good/bad, male/female, polyamorous/monogamous – we desperately want to know what the 'right' answer is, as if there's a universal template for happiness. As a consequence, most of the questions I'm asked to tackle on my sex blog point towards absolutes:

– Do women like anal sex? (They want a 'yes'.)
– What's the best chat-up line? (They want something akin to an 'abracadabra' that'll get anyone into their pants.)

– Who reads sex blogs more – men or women? (I'll tell you in a second.)

Some questions are easier to answer than others. The blog gets more visits now, so I have more data. I can answer questions like 'are people more likely to visit a porn site if you slag it off or if you praise it?' (Answer: slagging) and 'which sex toys are people most likely to search for and end up at my site?' (answer: butt plugs. You'd be surprised at how many questions I can ask to which 'butt plugs' are the answer). I'll never be able to answer questions one and two: they're far too subjective. I can no more tell you if women like buttsex than I can tell you whether women like Stilton, and if you're after a chat-up, the best I can do is tell you what would work on me ('Hey Sarah, would you like to watch me have a vigorous wank?'). But the men vs. women question is far more fun to answer, because it makes the point quite neatly.

Perhaps because I'm a female writer, or because I write dirty stories – more commonly labelled 'erotica' – people assume it's primarily read by women. In fact, 60% of my blog readers are men.

Sixty percent.

It feels so odd to have spent years shouting that 'sex isn't just for men!' only to find myself having to point out the seemingly obvious other side of the coin: sex blogs aren't just for women! These men probably wouldn't buy an erotic book with a swooning couple on the cover, but if you stick it on the Internet they'll rub one out just like the rest of us. I'd love it if everything were categorised based on preference, not gender, but as long as I need to make money, I'll have to care about these demographics. I get lots of requests from companies to put adverts on my blog, and it's interesting how many of them focus wholly on women. I get the odd escort agency that wants to target men, but sex toy companies and 'porn for women' sites will beg me for ad space under the assumption that my readers are mostly female. Some sex toy companies are surprised when I give them the (albeit not perfect) gender breakdown, and I can see why: for a long time sex toys and erotica have both been presented as the 'female' equivalents of jerking off to hardcore porn. A softer version of the bare-handed, manly wanking that guys do while watching *Anal Gangbang 4*. Obviously these assumptions are self-perpetuating – the more they're repeated the more people will tailor their products towards the stereotype, meaning all the *Anal Gangbangs* are shot with Mark in mind, and sex toys are labelled 'for her pleasure' and come in the shape of bunnies. Guys will see more ads featuring jiggling tits than shiny cock sheaths, and I see more vibrators than 'Hot DILFs in my area who really want to fuck'. We keep buying the stuff we're told to and it takes an age for us to realise that there's far more on offer. It's getting better, but even now, when things like masturbation sheaths for guys not only exist but look so goddamn futuristic and cool, few guys I know actually own one – many aren't aware they even exist. Female sex toys now come in such colours as 'not pink', but the marketing is still often taken from the 'Barbie' school of design. Don't despair, though – not only are there companies like Doxy making toys that don't assume we're scared of our vulvas, there's even a company called Bad Dragon which makes badass dildos shaped like dragon cocks. There are more sex toys for men than ever before, and even major porn sites have started recognising that straight women need to wank too. We're getting there.

Initially I was reluctant to run any ads at all – not just because I was nervous about the minefield of sex assumptions. On a practical level, I didn't want to send invoices with my real-life name on, or write reviews of sex toys that I wouldn't otherwise use. More importantly that I'm not even half as good at the sex toys thing as my other sex blogging colleagues. I can wax lyrical for hours about why lube is a lifesaver, or why anyone with a prostate should have a butt plug in their bedside drawer, but I don't have a huge sex toy collection of my own, or a drawer full of latex. I'm not great at big sex expos or shiny parties, where people arrive in spectacular outfits and spank each other on high-end bondage furniture. I like sordid frotting in corners and dirty trysts in alleyways. Fucking on the carpet at home until the skin on my knees is burned raw. The kind of fuck that makes him put his hand over my mouth to shush me in case the neighbours are listening. In those kinds of shags a set of anal beads may play a brief cameo, but it will never be the star of the show, so the sex I write about won't sell many buzzing pleasure products. I'm not saying my kind of sex is better, by the way: this isn't goths versus lip gloss again. To those who like decadence, shiny toys, sparkling thongs and huge PVC boots – good luck to you. I'll certainly be watching from the sidelines and weaving you into my fantasies later. It's just that I'll probably be wearing a jumper and wishing someone would turn the music down.

Eventually I did start running ads, partly because I like money and I need to eat things, but mainly because if you pick one company and get them to pay you, then you can hide behind them to avoid having to talk to others, and end up showing yourself up to be way less competent than they think you are. It's the equivalent of telling a hot guy you've got a boyfriend, so you never end up disappointing him with your sexual technique.

So I hide behind anonymity, sit in my jumper and worry over stats, only occasionally having to tackle the issue of how to sell lube when all I have to say about it is 'It's quite nice smeared on my cunt'. And it occurs to me that when it comes to the adverts, I'm stupid for trying to twist what I do just to fit what already exists. If I start reviewing lube brands like I give a flying fuck, I'm just squashing myself into a space I'll never be comfy in. Other sex bloggers do the review thing spectacularly, gathering toys and lubes and whips until their bedrooms are piled high, and they can give you every detail on the differences between each. There are plenty of others who focus on photos, fantasy writing, erotic art, or niche fetishes. If I try to emulate any one of them, I'm just slapping on pink lip gloss and pretending I'm not a goth.

Our obsession with these binaries is rarely stronger than when it comes to gender. The first question when people are born, or often before: is it a boy or a girl? Pink or blue? Beautiful or strong? Princess or astronaut? Then most of us sit in these boxes for the rest of our lives. But we're lucky to live in exciting times. My generation is probably the first to have proudly out transgender and genderqueer activists appearing regularly in mainstream media, telling everyone who'll listen that it's a lot more complicated than that. That what's in your pants doesn't dictate what's in your head. That gender and sexuality don't fall within a rigid binary, and life is far more interesting and exciting than a simple mosaic of pink and blue. It'd be ridiculous of me to pretend I'm an expert in this stuff: I'm still figuring a lot of it out myself. But in the process of learning about it I get to challenge my own assumptions – about what I like, why, and whether rejecting something at one end of the spectrum means I have to rush straight to the other end of it.

When I bring up the gender binary, there are usually people who pop up to explain that it's simply evolution: men have to be a certain way and women another, and there's nothing waffling lefties like me can do about it. What's more, there will always be some people who perfectly match their gender stereotype. Women who love shopping and weird-shaped mascara brushes. Guys who love football and can be relied on to forget anniversaries. There's nothing wrong with being one of these people, just as there's nothing wrong with being a teenage goth. But the fact that it's seen as binary encourages us to pick a side: you can either be male or female, girly or hard, femme or tomboy, but you *must* accessorise your outfit with your conviction that the other side is wrong.

A while ago there was a silly season incident in which a rumour went round the Internet that there was a lion loose in Essex. The story was total bullshit, but gave a fun afternoon's diversion for those of us looking for excuses not to do our real work. Unfortunately, alongside all the jokes about lions there was a deluge of extra sludge to wade through: the traditional piss-takes of 'Essex girls'. The stereotype about Essex girls is a heady mixture of misogyny and classism, wrapped up with a smug sense of superiority. Essex girls, so the story goes, are wannabe Barbies – they use fake tan and have acrylic nails. They wear short skirts and low-cut tops and they all want to be footballers' wives. They're thick. They're grotesque. They are – in short – inferior. When the lion was on the loose, my Twitter timeline – usually filled with worthy lefties explaining why women should be able to do whatever the fuck they please with their bodies, was suddenly filled with hateful jokes:

'There's a beast on the loose in Essex – long talons, massive hair, orange face. And there's a lion too!'

The jokes weren't being made by the usual brand of arsehole, they were being made by fluffy liberal types – the people who'd usually retweet or high-five me for posting about body hair or confidence. It made me want to throw a tantrum, shouting 'but you're supposed to be *on my side*!' If you agree that a woman has every right not to shave her armpits, then you have to be consistent and agree that she can if she wants to. You can't support a woman's right to physical autonomy if you subsequently spit on those who pick a look you don't personally like. You can't decide that the only way to rebel against a culture that tells us to preen is to hate on the people who want to. It makes no sense. If someone wants to stand next to me in my scruffy jeans, with legs they haven't shaved for two weeks, I'd love them to join me. I'll be here alongside hot muscular girls in dungarees and boxer shorts, girls in floral summer dresses and subtle how-does-she-achieve-that-look make-up. We'll join punks and goths and hipsters and Essex girls and people who are beach-body-ready by every possible definition of that phrase, but if this is going to work we have to *all* be welcome. It doesn't matter who anyone fancies, or whose style they'd personally steal, it's about crushing the idea that you have to have a 'style' in the first place. That you have to pick a side and then snipe from the sidelines at people who choose differently.

It's hard to shake the feeling that there's something about each of us that we need to 'fix' or address before we become proper grown-ups. Wipe off that awful black lipstick, put on a sensible outfit and go get yourself a husband. It's tempting to see this as a war between factions. Right/wrong, good/bad, conform/rebel. If I could talk to my teenage self, apart from giving her a decent black lipstick to save wasting the eyeliner, I'd give her a bit of advice: challenging stereotypes isn't about just 'doing the opposite', it's about respecting every choice equally, including the ones you wouldn't pick yourself. Teenage goths, happy housewives, Essex girls, whoever: you're either with us or against us, but you can't just be with *some* of us.

When Love Requires Sacrifice

(chastityproject.com)

Me: What's the most embarrassing tattoo you could get, do you reckon?
Him: I could get your face... tattooed on my face.

I always imagine registry offices to be fairly bland places: bare walls and simple rows of chairs that look like they've been borrowed from the job centre down the road. Guests tapping their watches in the hope that the quick fire ceremony will be even quicker and they can get on with the drinking afterwards. It's not like that here though – the registry is pretty and warm and there's a feeling of genuine excitement. The odd elderly relative makes pointed jokes that 'it's about bloody time', but no one takes it in the nagging spirit it's intended. When the registrar calls us through, she beams with genuine pleasure: as if she doesn't do this 20 times a day, and hasn't yet become bored of people using the same old song to walk up the aisle to ('Thousand Years' by Christina Perri, in case you're interested). Not one of us glances at a watch, or worries whether the bride will be on time: she's here already, slightly tipsy from breakfast champagne, in a bright red dress and dazzling smile.

Not *me*, bloody hell: my mum. My brilliant, pisshead, hopelessly-in-love mum. Less than four steps up the aisle, she starts to cry, which means I lose a bet with my sister – I had a quid on her lasting until the vows. My stepdad starts to blub the second she walks in.

Yeah, I know – my stepdad cheated. Bad guy, right? In the story he should get comeuppance, not wedding cake. By all rights my mother should have had an epiphany, tipped red wine over him in public while an Aretha Franklin tune swelled in the background, before sashaying off into the arms of someone chiselled and witty. She didn't, although (because my mum is fucking *dynamite*) it wasn't for a lack of offers. A week after my stepdad had slumped off to see what he could make of his mid-life love affair, my mum had two of her long-lost exes lined up and begging for dates. She explained to me over a glass of rosé (which signals a much happier break-up than gin), 'It turns out I'm at exactly the age where people get divorced. I had my first one far too early, but now *everyone's* at it.' We leant against the wall in my back garden and smoked cigarettes – what had initially felt like the end of the world now felt like the start of a party.

'What do you think I should do?' she asked, as if our roles had been reversed and I – now 'settled' – was better qualified to decide. My mum's ideas about happy ever after had packed their bags and left along with my stepdad, and

I quite liked the hormonal teenage girl who'd moved in to take their place. 'Should I go on a date with either of them?'

I tried so hard to be restrained – to think about what a sensible person would suggest when one of their parents has just been ripped to shreds by the love of their life, and is staring at two potentially unwise rebound flings.

'Phone them now. Phone *both of them* now.'

'It's two in the morning.'

'OK. Phone both of them *tomorrow*.'

I poured some more wine, and she told me how she met each of them, and we spent the rest of the night trying to imagine what it would be like if either managed to live up to that nostalgic promise.

Don't press play on the Aretha Franklin track just yet, though. My stepdad had something those other guys didn't. In fact, a whole bunch of 'somethings' that on their own seem unimportant, but swell into significance when you put them together: 20 years' worth of shared memories. Thousands of evenings spent with each others' children, hundreds of Sundays playfully fighting over the weekend supplements, Friday nights drinking wine at the piano and swearing at the other one's fuck-ups. You can hate someone's cheating, but still love them for everything else. When my stepdad came back (I said my mum's dynamite, *of course* he came back) the tipsy fantasies about other guys couldn't compete with the mountain of memories.

After the reception we pile into a minibus and head to the pub. My stepdad pops champagne and pours Mum a glass, before putting his arm around her shoulders and kissing her forehead, and I wonder what he's thinking. His eyes are red from crying and he looks older than he did a year ago.

They struggled to get over the cheating and if you catch me in an honest moment I'll tell you they still do. He didn't just make a swift, horny mistake – he walked away from their life together, saying not just 'I love her' but 'I don't love *you*'. No matter how many tears of joy he sheds at the altar, having realised he actually does, they won't wash away the fact that once he thought he didn't. Did my mum make the right decision? It's not up to me, any more than it's up to her if I choose to marry Mark. I do know that she's happy right now, kissing him through giggles at another shared joke. I know she won't be happy every day – she'll have her moments of certainty that the whole thing will end, just like I do. I wonder if she smiled when he proposed, or if she narrowed her eyes suspiciously as I would, asking why he thought that a marriage would succeed where a simple 'I love you' might not. Perhaps she liked the idea of walking down the aisle, because she realised none of her rebellious children would be saying 'I do' any time soon, and she fancied a bit of a party. Maybe in that moment the most romantic thing she did was say 'yes' to something just because it made him happy.

There's nothing like a wedding to inspire you to romance, is there? Let's have another go at this 'romance' thing and see if I can do something nice for Mark. I'll start small and we'll work up, because the pull of the rom-com is strong, and I'd like to end on something dramatic.

I bake him a cake. Don't laugh: it's a *really* good cake. All chocolate decadence and gooey (undercooked) centre. Raspberry coulis splattered on top, dripping through the layers. This isn't a cake you can slice and eat nicely: this is a cake that's messy like a lubed-up hallway fuck. A cake you tear at with your bare fists before shoving the sweetness into someone's mouth, watching them grin through smears of icing. It's a good cake, OK? It's Valentine's Day, too, which means that even if the cake does look a little wonky, and the icing is a bit runnier than I'd ideally like, the day makes the gesture more symbolic. All I have to do now is ice some words on the top. Some phrase or saying that I know will touch Mark right in his soppy heart and make him want to squeeze me with his big hands, whisper 'I love you too', before sliding his hand down the back of my jeans and squeezing my arse so hard his fingers slip deep into my butt crack. Of all the things Mark likes, he likes Netflix the most: Netflix, pizza, blow jobs – the magic trio that fits neatly into his life plan of 'Living every day as if mild enjoyment is all you've ever wished for'. What's more, today might be Valentine's Day, but it's also the day that Netflix release season two of a drama series we're both obsessed with. One in which a slightly odd, sexually-charged couple work together to take over the world. So I choose that, and when Mark comes home he's greeted by a pile of messy baking tins and a cake that shakily wishes him 'Happy House of Cards Day'.

'I love it,' he grins, grabbing me around the shoulders and pulling me into a hug. 'You're the *best*.'

Level one complete: on to level two.

I was due to go away for a week with my sister. Mark was simultaneously sad and delighted that he couldn't come: sad because he'd miss me, delighted because it gave him time to catch up on all the Xbox games he'd missed while we were reclaiming my sexual mojo. His cute apology cards ('Sorry I called you a prick!') are one of my favourite things, but I assume my own attempts at romance should be unique. After a quick Google for 'original romance ideas' I came across the idea of a treasure hunt. It wasn't an awesome hunt; please don't mistake me for someone competent. I'd have loved to lay a complex trail of riddles, which had him puzzling for just the right length of time before he lit upon a sexy memory which would lead him to the right place:

'My first word's a city, my second is "tube"

I once sucked you off here, and you touched my boob!'

(The clue, naturally, would lead him to the rather misleadingly titled 'Oxford Tube', which is actually a fucking *bus*. On this *bus*, the only entertainment when you're returning to London late at night is to have an illicit liaison on the back seat. Mark covered my head with a coat while I pretended to sleep on his lap. Then I took his dick slowly into my mouth, using my tongue around the head to keep him hard for half the journey, until he finally gave in somewhere around the M40 and pumped a torrent of frustrated spunk right down the back of my throat. It costs just under £20 return, and I'd give it five stars if the Wi-Fi had worked).

While I'd have loved to send him on a London-wide goose chase, I remembered that romantic gestures shouldn't be about what *I* want (to get Mark out of the house so he doesn't die of rickets while I'm gone); they had to be about him. So I made the 'clues' as direct as he was ('Tomorrow's clue: in the drawer in the cellar where we keep all the fucking magnets') and sprinkled sweets liberally in each hiding place. I popped the first clue on the kitchen counter, picked up my backpack, and rushed off to the airport, imagining his delighted face when he opened the first one and realised what was in store.

To keep his expectations suitably low, the first one read:

'I love you so much I put some effort into doing something. Tomorrow's clue is in the lube box.'

Over the week, they built up to more specific affectionate pronouncements such as:

'Without you my life would be at least 35% shitter. Next clue's in the bathroom cabinet.'

and

'You've got a lovely cock. Next clue's at the back of your pants drawer.'

For the grand finale, I'd stashed loads more sweets and I wanted to accompany it with a correspondingly large declaration of love. Still struggling to say anything genuinely warm without sounding a bit sarcastic, I fumbled for a way to sum up what Mark was to me. 'You're my...' hmm. 'Baby' is too cute. 'Other half' has nice connotations of togetherness but implies that I can't be complete on my own – apart from the fact that I couldn't write it, I know Mark would struggle to *believe* it. 'You're my rock' will get him worried that I'm about to have another breakdown. 'Darling'? Vomit. 'Sweet'? Double-vomit. 'Favourite'? Makes him sound like a Liquorice Allsort.

Eventually it hit me. The miracle of Mark's patience, and his goodness and his tendency to stay despite everything. That I can't help but love him. No matter what I do or who I meet, no one will ever compete with the steadfast, nerdy, reliably brilliant Mark. So I let *Doctor Who* say it for me:

'You are my Rory.'

He texts me to tell me he cried, and we are equally disgusted at the soppy twats we've become.

I'm getting better at romance when I stop worrying so much about it. What's the next step – a marriage proposal, perhaps? A super-personalised one, which speaks to something Mark loves deeply, and demonstrates my willingness to compromise on the whole white dress/aisle/patriarchal tradition of marriage that my teenage-goth self would rage against. Here's the shortlist:

1. Coffee. I could train as a barista (not properly, just enough that I can pull off the neat trick where they draw things in the foam), then present Mark with a perfectly made coffee. I think I've got it down now – I know all the things that are important. Via the medium of teasing him about being a coffee snob I am now aware of which beans are best, and how important it is to freshly grind them (we're on our third aluminium coffee grinder now – those things aren't as robust as you think, especially when you get an idea in your head and it turns out that using an electric drill to try and grind the beans faster only ends up shaving the metal). I don't know the difference between a flat white and a latte because nobody does (the Emperor's naked, people: I'm calling it) but I *do* know why it's important not to scald the milk. If I learned how to prepare the perfect cup of coffee, as a final flourish I could write 'Mark, will you marry me?' in the foam. Or, perhaps more realistically 'Marry?', because coffee cups are small and wonky writing is hard to read.

2. Chocolate. It's a bit similar to the treasure hunt idea, but that one seemed to work. How about I doctor a Cadbury's advent calendar, so that in the lead up to Christmas Mark gets a letter each day along with a delicious chocolate? December 1st: 'W', December 2nd: 'I'. December 3rd: 'L', and so on, until on December 24th the entire message can be read in full, through crumpled foil and torn cardboard: 'WILL YOU MARRY ME?' That's only 18 characters, though. Even if I added a filler word ('prick' has the requisite five letters, for instance), the game would be up by the time he got to the end of 'you'. The chocolate would be a hit, but I think Mark would prefer it with a twist ending, such as 'WILL YOU...' (pause for excitement on day nine) '...BUY ME A PONY?' Come to think of it, that's almost exactly the right number. I should do that anyway. Don't show him this book.
3. Computery things. I know that's vague. If Mark had the decency to work in an comprehensible job I could be more specific. I understand security updates and printer jams, and how to install the new Windows then reinstall the old version of Windows because the new one is inevitably rubbish. But what Mark does with computers is far too complex, no matter how hard I frown and concentrate when he tries to explain what a 'stack overflow' is, or why Java is not the same thing as Java*script*. He's keen for me to learn, but only because he feels selfish keeping all the computery joy to himself. Like he's eating the best biscuits out of the tin and if I'd only have a nibble on one of the better chocolate ones my eyes would be open and he'd have given me a share of his happiness. It's not true, any more than it's true

that he'd love reading my novels, but perhaps that can be my sacrifice for him. I'll spend however many hours it takes to build a rudimentary app, then sneakily install it on his phone so the next time he goes to launch his email, his screen explodes in a shower of hearts and flowers, and plays something cheese-laden like 'Marry You' by Bruno Mars.

I'm actually considering this last idea as we sit on the train, on our way to visit Lucy and meet her new baby.

'How easy is it to make an app?' I ask. He stares at me, quite rightly, like I've just asked him to fax me an email. 'It depends,' he says very slowly and clearly 'on what you want the app to do. Do you want me to help you build an app?'

'No.' I say sulkily, and stare out of the window. For fuck's sake – how am I supposed to do something nice for him in secret when all he wants to do is *help*?'

When we arrive at Lucy's the baby is as adorable as you'd expect. Tiny and pink and beautiful, swaddled in reusable linen nappies and clutching a Freecycled quilt. I marvel at her teeny fingers before passing her on to Mark, whereupon she falls fast asleep on his chest. Lucy is perfect in all the right ways. She doesn't coo and say the baby's changed her life, or that the birth was miraculous. Covered in that fine layer of yellowish spit that marks all new parents, she explains how traumatic the birth was, with colourful detail on a couple of medical procedures that I'd rather never have heard of. When we quiz her on the next part – the actual motherhood – Lucy explains matter-of-factly:

'It's not what I expected.' Her husband nods. They're presenting a deliciously united front. 'It's nice, sure, but hard.' Mark cradles the baby's head in his hands – big hands, designed for safe cradling and never dropping stuff. I fidget and ask Lucy to elaborate.

'Everyone says you're just hit with this lightning bolt of pure love. And I haven't had that yet.'

Mark's looking at the baby but I know he's listening carefully. He expects the lightning bolt, and the knowledge that it doesn't always appear might upset him.

'Don't get me wrong, I'm sure some people get it,' Lucy explains. 'And I love her, of course I love her. But right now I'm aching and sore and covered in... stuff... and it's all I can do to stay awake.'

Maybe this cheery acceptance of her flaws is why it seems like Lucy has everything right: she ticks the boxes but refuses to behave like ticking boxes is the only thing worth doing. She's the first of my close friends to have a baby and she's one of the only people I know who speaks like this about babies. Not 'Oh you *must*!' or 'You'll change your mind' but 'Here's what I think: make up your own'. When we hand the baby back to the flustered parents, she opens her eyes. She's on the brink of tears – sleep? Hunger? About-to-shit-her-nappy? No idea. My mum says women tend to know these things by instinct, but I'm stumped.

'Sorry. Is she sad because I woke her up?' asks Mark, quickly adding 'Hungry? Needs changing?' He's desperate to get the answer right, perhaps to show that he'd be great at this parenting thing himself. We look to Lucy and her husband to see what their instincts tell them.

'Not a clue,' Lucy's husband replies cheerfully, taking the angry bundle of muslin out of Mark's hands.

'Could be anything,' adds Lucy, before starting the cycle of feed/burp/change/cuddle that might help shed some light on it. Mark watches them intently, trying to learn so that next time she cries he'll be able to help. Having held the baby for all of five minutes he's fallen a teeny bit in love with her, and – like his offer of help with my ill-thought-out app – all he wants is to help her too.

Maybe if I want to do something truly nice for Mark, I should make a proper sacrifice: say yes to something just because it makes him happy. Help him do what he loves to do best: hug. Cuddle. Love. Help. Maybe the most romantic thing I can do is to give him a family.

10 Scientifically Proven Ways To Be Incredibly Happy

(inc.com)

- He watches a child smearing food on his dad's jumper -
Him: The problem with kids though, is if you do *have them, you can't have anything else that's nice.*

It's Wednesday again. No matter how much navel-gazing you do, you'll always come back round to a Wednesday. The day of the week least likely to contain life-changing developments and, therefore, the one that most deserves attention.

This Wednesday, I'm with Adam.

I won't lie: he's still my type. Still fidgets in his seat, long-limbed and twitching with eagerness to tell me his latest story. Dark eyes sparkling as he – oh god, *the hottest thing* – builds to a punchline that's genuinely funny. In my head I write a blog post praising the curve of his smile when he used to kiss me, or each detail of every one of his knuckles – how he'd bury them in my cunt when I begged. It shouldn't be sexual any more though – we're mates. Not friends: *mates*. Competitive, boisterous and ever-so-slightly-wary-of-each-other. Perhaps the wariness is only in my head, coming as it does from the fact that I can't look at him without wanting to touch. I sit near him, aware of every movement of each of my limbs – holding myself stiffly so I don't accidentally brush against him. If I cross my legs and my foot touches his, I have to fidget to cover for the fact that I jumped. He's still my type. Mark and I could ensconce ourselves in a comfortable suburbia from now until forever and still Adam could pop up next to my deathbed and have me dripping lust into my granny knickers. We talk about his girlfriend and his job and his plans for the future and I forget to be annoyed that he hasn't asked about Mark. When we say goodbye at the end of the evening, the hug is exactly one crotch-throb longer than it should be and I inhale that same sexy scent of his neck before he dashes to catch the last train.

On the way home, I manage to hold on to that slightly guilty lust until the second I check my phone. Then the lust switches, as it always does, for anxiety. A blog post went live this evening, and it's started a kerfuffle. Where 'kerfuffle' is the mild word I use to try and calm the racing panic that washes over me when I see comments that start with 'bullshit' and end with a plosive 'bitch'. Just as every thud of lust makes me wonder if I'll fuck things up with Mark, so each angry comment feels like the one that will bring my blog crashing down and my name into the open. When I explain how I stay anonymous, I rarely remember to list the most important trick of all: try to make people like you. It's impossible, of course, like chasing eternal happiness. You'll never make *everyone* like you on the Internet – even if you only ever talk about kittens and bacon, you'll still have vegans grabbing pitchforks. But you can *try*. You can try so hard it makes your stomach churn and your veins throb. So I worry and smile and try, and run through everything with a fine toothcomb, then when people kick off in the comments I say 'I see what you're saying' or 'Let's agree to disagree'. Because no matter how many bulletproof panels I surround myself with, how many layers of fake names and friends who plant secrets to lead people off the scent, the most useful tool in my anonymity arsenal is preventing people from *wanting* to find out. While I'm 'Girl on the Net' I'm mysterious and interesting, a potential rampaging sex kitten who they may meet one dark and sexy night. As soon as I'm outed I shrink back to Sarah: tedious human with shit music taste, an erratic libido and a tendency to cry at John Lewis adverts. So I play nice and I swallow some angry words, then I fuck up and forget and piss people off anyway. That's when it's time to cross my fingers and hope no one is pissed off enough to find me.

I swipe left on my phone to try and clear all the notifications then hurry home to Mark, breathing as well as I can when my lungs are burning and I'm trying to squeeze the panic out of my mind. It builds, as it was bound to, and Mark helps, as he always does.

We try to have sex.

And the word 'try' makes me want to weep. What worked an hour ago, when I was sitting across from Adam, is now utterly broken, and the shag I wanted to bring home to Mark peters out into a cuddle.

'Fuck off, I *love* a good cuddle,' he says, as I mumble apologies to try and make him feel better. 'Don't worry about it.'

But I'm pissed, and I'm tired, so I do. My heart's still beating like it's trying to fucking kill me, my brain doesn't work and my cunt's let me down and those five words make me limp with misery: 'We tried to have sex'. The way that simply trying feels like failure. It's a far cry from 'we fucked', and it's nothing like happy ever after.

Most of the questions I get asked on the blog, by people who are kind enough to think I'll know the answer, can be boiled down to one thing: how can I be happy? I don't know the answer any better than they do, but I chase the same thing, asking friends and family to give me some kind of magic formula. Dave's response is 'Move to Thailand' – it's always 'Move to Thailand' – and I like the significance of that. It's big and comfortable and solid, because it's never going to happen. My mum, naturally, says 'Grandchildren' with an excited grin. My dad gives financial advice and tells me that if I get married, he'd be happy to put a marquee up on his lawn. Claire is more helpful, which is surprising given that she's most of the way through a bottle of prosecco when I ask her:

'Just accept that you love Mark and you're basically happy already.'

'So what's next?'

'Does there have to be a "next"?'

I raise my eyebrows. For *her* there'd be a next. She's just been telling me about her new boyfriend – he's ticked the tall, dark, handsome boxes, as well as the rather vital 'shags like a dog on viagra' box, yet even a mere three dates in she's already considering the 'next'.

'Is it shallow of me if I dump him because he doesn't laugh at my jokes?'

'Maybe it's because...'

'...my jokes aren't funny. I know. But I'm not sure he has a sense of humour *at all*.'

'Probably not a keeper. It's not that all guys have to be funny, just that *yours* needs to be.'

She agrees, and tells me that, post-divorce, she's become far stricter about her criteria: husband number two will be funny, smart, earning roughly the same as she does to avoid any arguments, and will definitely want children one day. The guys she meets are different in many ways (jobs, looks, quantity of fruit they sculpt in their spare time), but the kids issue helps her to sort them more easily. I envy her certainty, which is more tempting than an infinite list of 'maybes'. Maybe I *would* have children, if Mark really wanted them. Maybe I *will* change my mind one day, and have to swallow an entire humble pie when I tell my mum. For Claire, there's no such thing as a 'maybe', but for Mark and I it seems like the only answer that has ever made sense.

Lucy's solution fits her perfectly: it's haphazardly practical, concrete decisions that still leave wiggle room for fuck-ups along the way. How does she do it? How does she *decide*?

'I'm not entirely sure I have, mate.' She whips out a boob and starts feeding the baby. 'If you're waiting for some kind of revelation, you'll be waiting till you're dead.'

'But what about the baby?' She shrugs and the baby temporarily loses her nipple, so she quickly adjusts before the wailing begins.

'We decided we wanted to try for kids and I think the phrase "try" helps out a bit – you're not really making a decision, you're just *starting* to make a decision and then BAM – you're pregnant. Even when I was as big as a house and eating curries to try and get labour to start, I still wasn't 100% sure about motherhood.'

'So what do you do?'

'You just... get on with it.' She's getting a bit exasperated now and I can see why. In my head – and probably on this page – I sound like one of those nagging kids who keep asking why the sky is blue. 'Do you think *I* never wonder what my life would be like if I weren't married? Or fancy anyone else? Obviously I do. But that's good. If I *never* wondered about any of that then what I have wouldn't be valuable, it'd just be a thing that happened to me. I love my life and I love being here, and the way I show that is that I make the *choice* to do it.' I get what she's saying – love isn't just something that you establish with a grand gesture, which then lasts forever, it's an active choice that you keep making every day. What's been confusing me about it is that, while I've made the decision to be with Mark, I still worry that he's shackled himself to me. That he's made his life smaller by sharing it with someone who will never be as good as he is. His ambitions of children are more significant than my dreams of a writing shed and shag-friendly sofas, so I assume his decision to stay must be more significant too. It's that self-hating narcissism again – *my* choice isn't relevant but *yours* is monumental. And in this case, it's not my choice to make.

'What if,' I start, tentatively, 'we *never* have a baby?'

'Then we'd never have a baby.'

'Would you be sad?"

'I don't know.'

Long pause. I think this conversation would be improved if we were having it in the rain, or at an airport departure lounge before one of us flew off to Australia. Mark reckons:

'This would be a better conversation if we had pizza.'

I order a pizza.

'You know,' he says. 'If we had a baby we probably couldn't eat this much pizza.'

'Why?'

'Got to set an example. Eat... broccoli and stuff.'

'True.'

'And we probably couldn't afford pizza because we'd have bought baby things.'

We sit in silence for a while, and I tell him what he already knows:

'I don't think I ever want one.'

'I know.'

'But if you really want one, you have time to find some-one else.'

'I know.'

More silence. God, he's right about the pizza – at least it would fill the pauses.

'So why haven't you?'

'What, found someone else?'

'Yeah.'

'Christ, you're an arsehole.'

He drags me into a horizontal sofa hug and we lie there for a while. He breathes in and I breathe out, and I push myself into his chest that's at just the right temperature for a cuddle.

'Listen,' he explains. 'Yes, I would like to have a baby. But would I like to have a baby at the expense of all the other stuff? Probably not. All the things I like doing every day: eating pizza, getting high, going to see that Matt Damon film three times because it's awesome, getting drunk and counting pennies. All the little things...'

'But the *big* things...'

'Sssh. The little things are only fun because I can do them *with you*. I wouldn't expect the big things to be any different. You're obsessed with the big things.'

'Am I?'

'Yes. Just shut up and enjoy this.'

'So no baby?'

'Don't think of it as "no baby", think of it as "unlimited pizza."'

If this were a rom-com the delivery driver would have arrived right then – perfect timing, to highlight Mark's point. But this is real life, so it didn't.

'Half an hour before pizza gets here,' Mark said, pulling casually at my shirt. 'This. Take it off.'

There's no grand finale for Mark and I – we don't get married. We don't have children. We don't split up. Neither of us runs off into the sunset and given that we live in London we're more likely to slope off into the drizzle anyway. But while it looks the same on the surface, beneath it's very different. This day, unlike the one at the start of the book, isn't something we fell into: it's a choice. I've been worried because in an ideal world, we'd both want to tick the same boxes (marriage, children, none of the above), but in reality we've both ticked the one that really matters: we want to be together. I can no more tell you how this story ends than I can tell you what love is, explain what counts as cheating, or detail how you can blow someone's mind in bed. We spend our lives writing and rewriting our own love stories, occasionally hoping for climaxes or scribbling out chapters we regret. Along the way people ask us for progress reports: Do you have a boyfriend? Are you married yet? Do you have kids? As with the sex blog questions, it's always tempting to offer an answer – or at the very least some advice that's based on what works for me. But if I try to persuade you that your own path should follow mine, then I'm no better than the people who nag you about wedding bells.

Love, for you, might mean suburban Wednesdays. It might mean an open relationship. It might mean fondue, fruit sculpture or a shared passion for upcycling. Your love may be a bolt from the blue, a slow realisation, or a plot-filled rollercoaster of uncertainty.

So we wake up on Wednesdays and I grind coffee, we save up for sofas and we talk about kids: all the suburban things that used to scare me. We also get drunk and ride bikes and fuck loudly, and dream of all the things we could achieve as just the two of us. We come up with ridiculous ways to trick our mates into thinking we're magic and count pennies on the living room floor. Of all the myths we're told about relationships, perhaps the most frustrating one is that there's a correct answer and when you've chosen it you're done. That's it. Hand in your work and ride off into the sunset. Maybe that's why we often feel the need for a big romantic gesture – a decision to be with someone forever needs a correspondingly huge announcement, with rings and champagne and a viral YouTube video, and a party your gran can get drunk at.

But if Mark and I don't make a big decision, we get to make the little ones over and over – that's half the fun. I choose to be with Mark and I get to make that choice every day – each time I refuse a shag from a stranger, come home drunk with new sex toys, or bake a crap cake for Valentine's Day. Every day that my heart beats with panic and I feel like the world's going to end, when Mark takes me in his big arms and holds me and I realise that it's *not* a trap – I've chosen to be here because it's the place that makes me happiest.

Epilogue

From the dirtiest fucks to the cheesiest romantic moments, whenever I write about Mark I get asked the same question: how does he feel about this? I figure here is as good a place to answer it as any. I panic that I never write him well enough. That just by trying to capture him on paper I've turned him into a caricature: a paler, weaker version of the Mark who's with me now. You see only 1% of him, because to paint the whole picture is impossible. When it's a tiny character or a quick scene – Lucy, Claire, Dave, my parents – the skewed perspective doesn't matter as much. I don't think they'll mind if I use these snippets, as long as I point out it's not the full story. But when the whole book is about Mark? It matters.

What does he think?

As I write this, he's curled up in the living room reading through the first draft, occasionally adding comments or pointing to his crotch when he gets to a horny bit. He sometimes offers suggestions if there's a section I've struggled with, or chips in a new swear word if I've used too many 'pricks'. He cries when he gets to the part about the doctor and when he reads chapters on cheating he tells me it'll all be fine. He smiles at the baby stuff, laughs at his jokes and when he's finished, he hugs me.

Me: What do you think? I still need to end on a romantic gesture.

Him: What?

Me: You know, something significant that shows how much I love you.

Him: Fuck's sake, dickhead – you just wrote me a whole book.

Acknowledgements

As soon as you take something from a blog into a book, it becomes a group effort, which can potentially be utterly terrifying. So massive thanks to Emily Thomas at Blink for turning 'scary' into 'exciting', and to everyone at Blink for all their hard work and support. Also a huge thank you to my agent, Lorella Belli, who is amazing to work with, exceptionally patient when I'm stressed and eagle-eyed at spotting when I accidentally advertise Wetherspoons.

Massive thanks to 'Claire', 'Lucy', and my amazing best mate 'Dave', as well as other people behind fake names who have let me use their words of wisdom. I'm sorry if I've not done you justice, as I'm sure I haven't. That goes double for the guys who let me write about them: 'Michael', 'Owen' and especially 'Adam'.

Stuart Taylor, who illustrates my blog so beautifully – I genuinely can't thank you enough for all you've done. Also all the fantastic guest bloggers who share slices of their own lives and give me more reason to keep blogging. People who have helped me understand a hell of a lot more than I did when I started: Pandora Blake, Justin Hancock, Emma Podmore, Petra Joy, Ruby Kiddell, Cara Sutra, Molly Moore, DomSigns, Meg John Barker and so many others. Supportive mates who've given me more than a helping hand: Dean Burnett, Nate Crowley, G, O, Martin, Liam, Internet Jen and Company-X-Jen, and especially my fantastic 'boss' Jon. Thanks also to the people on Twitter who helped me with my maths – Dr J, @xabl, @Andrew_Taylor and others. All those I've inevitably missed off this list, for which I'm incredibly sorry.

It feels weird for a 'thanks' page to include people who haven't read the book, but I'm incredibly grateful to my amazing family, who support me without ever asking too many questions. My sister who saves the world and is my personal hero, my mum who is extraordinary, my brother who is far cooler than me, my stepdad who taught me that people can be brilliant and flawed at the same time, and my dad, stepbrother and stepmum. I'm lucky to have all of you, thank you for not reading.

We live in a capitalist country in which things aren't possible without money, so thanks also to the people who pay my bills so I don't starve, as well as everyone who has supported my blog – commented, offered advice, linked and shared and corrected me when I have (frequently) been wrong. I look forward to being wrong some more in the future.

And Mark, of course. Thank you for putting up with my grumpy writing moods – I owe you something and a pizza.